AIDS
A PILGRIMAGE
TO HEALING

R.P. Hardy

Read - 30 Nov 1993

AIDS
A PILGRIMAGE TO HEALING

Peter B. Todd

A GUIDE FOR HEALTH PROFESSIONALS, CLERGY, EDUCATORS AND CARERS

MILLENNIUM BOOKS
DAVID LOVELL

First published in 1992 by
Millennium Books
an imprint of E.J. Dwyer (Australia) Pty Ltd
3/32–72 Alice Street
Newtown NSW 2042
Australia

in association with
David Lovell Publishing
308 Victoria Street
Brunswick Victoria 3056

Copyright © 1992 Peter B. Todd
This book is copyright. Apart from any fair dealing for
the purposes of private study, research, criticism or
review, as permitted under the Copyright Act, no part
may be reproduced by any process without written
permission. Inquiries should be addressed to the publisher.

National Library of Australia
Cataloguing-in-Publication data

Todd, Peter B. (Peter Bryan), 1944– .
  AIDS, a pilgrimage to healing.

  Bibliography
  Includes index.
  ISBN 0 85574 902 4.

  1. AIDS (Disease) – Psychological aspects. 2. HIV (Viruses) –
  Psychological aspects. 3. Mental healing. 4. AIDS (Disease) –
  Religious aspects. I. Title.

362.1969792

Cover design by Stanley Wong
Typeset in Palatino 11/12 pt by Graphicraft Typesetters Ltd, Hong Kong
Printed in Australia by The Book Printer

Distributed in Canada by:

Meakin and Associates
Unit 17
81 Auriga Drive
NEPEAN, ONT K2E 7Y5
Ph: (613) 226 4381

Distributed in Ireland and the U.K. by:

Columba Book Service
93 The Rise
Mount Merrion
BLACKROCK CO. DUBLIN
Ph: (01) 283 2954

Distributed in the United States by:

Morehouse Publishing
871 Ethan Allen Highway
RIDGEFIELD CT 06877
Ph: (203) 431 3927

FOREWORD

In July 1990, Australia's population was reported to be in excess of seventeen million, with somewhere between 60–90,000 people estimated to be HIV infected. Recent statistics have indicated the presence of 16,000 cases of HIV antibody positive status, confirmed by actual testing or screening. When one adds to that figure the partners, spouses, lovers, families, friends, professional health care workers, clergy and community support networks, we have an ever widening number of people directly involved in the HIV/AIDS pandemic. Forecasts of the continued spread of the virus are chilling. WHO estimates a global population of HIV positive men, women and children to exceed 25 million by 2000. The horizon does indeed look bleak. In Australia alone, more than 2000 people have already died, with an annual mortality of about 700.

So why another book on AIDS? Bookshops have rows of titles dedicated to almost every angle on the epidemic. However, when one looks closely, one lacuna becomes obvious. To date, very little, if anything at all, has been written on the psycho-spiritual dimensions of AIDS. Peter Todd's book is an attempt to remedy this deficiency.

The image of pilgrimage is one that is familiar to people of most cultures and religions. It suggests a journey towards a place of special rest and replenishment. Traditionally, pilgrimages were made to holy places associated with particularly significant people or events. Jerusalem, Rome and Mecca spring to mind as places well known as pilgrim cities. There has always been another dimension to pilgrimage—that of an inner pilgrimage. This inner pilgrimage is a journey towards the centre of our humanity, a journey into the soul.

Perhaps such language is odd by our highly 'sophisticated' technical and empirical standards. Yet today, unlike any previous era, the cry for meaning rings loudly throughout the world. Human beings living with HIV/AIDS are confronted with questions of mortality, morality, identity, acceptance and faith. It can often be an overwhelming experience.

The image of pilgrimage is one of gradual progression, moving at a regular, even relaxed pace, towards the holy place. Pilgrims have time to reflect upon their relationship with themselves, the world and with God. The pilgrim knows that the journey will have moments of trial and hardship, but alongside that will be equally vivid moments of enlightenment, empowerment and healing. For people living with HIV/AIDS, the pilgrimage of AIDS can be one that allows a renaissance of life in the face of threatening death.

Peter Todd's contribution to this pilgrimage consists of wide experience in psychotherapy and group and face-to-face counseling, as well as his own personal journey from darkness into light. In this book, Todd seeks to place mental and spiritual approaches to healing on a scientific level, using experience in the field of breast cancer to find a common point in therapeutic work with people who are HIV positive. Another unarticulated area in this regard is the use of symbol and ritual in healing. Todd places before us quite compelling premises for the acceptance of these often neglected expressions of that which is beyond the merely empirical, as vibrant and energetic sources of healing and enlightenment. Quite clearly, there emerges a compelling argument to include and incorporate the religious dimension of human experience with the scientific approaches to HIV/AIDS. We are left in no doubt that 'new age quackery' has no place here!

Todd re-echoes Elisabeth Kübler-Ross' *AIDS: The Ultimate Challenge*, where she throws down the gauntlet to the world. Unless we are willing to learn, or to re-learn, how to love unconditionally the person living and dying with AIDS, and thus allow *ourselves* to experience healing, as well as offer healing, we shall become a crippled, introspective people. We shall slowly die of a spiritual AIDS that will have consequences that reach far beyond the gay community, the IV drug users, prostitutes and others deemed 'socially inferior.'

What one realizes, in the face of HIV/AIDS, is the truth that we are all pilgrims, all on the journey towards that place of healing and wholeness. This book does not purport to claim a 'cure' for AIDS. What it does offer is the opportunity to use the riches of our common humanity in all its fulness, to re-discover the treasures that all human beings have within them. It is the pilgrimage to the great healing of discovering within the person living with AIDS the face of God. And perhaps we too shall discover the same face within ourselves.

Finally, Todd includes a challenge to the churches. As vehicles of communicating the healing and loving presence of God, our faith communities can provide havens and places of acceptance, tolerance and unconditional love. This book is a timely reminder that human beings are more than machines or objects. Todd invites us to go beyond what we so often see as limits, to risk discovering a new world, a new creation, a newness of life that we can scarce imagine.

> I have come that you may have life,
> and have it to the full!
>
> I tell you solemnly,
> in as much as you did this to these
> the least of my brothers and sisters,
> you did it to me.

Fr Paul O'Shea

CONTENTS

FOREWORD   Fr Paul O'Shea   v
PREFACE   Professor Anne Daniel   1
INTRODUCTION   The Miracle of Wholeness   5

Part One
THE ASCENT OF HOLISM

1   Revolutions in Understanding and Caring   9
2   The Origins of Holism and Psychosomatics   15
3   Psychoneuroimmunology: Emotions,
    Immunity and Disease   21

Part Two
RAISING CONSCIOUSNESS

4   A Holistic or Biopsychosocial Model of AIDS   31
5   Therapies: How Might We Modify
    Immunity and Illness?   38
6   A Long Night's Journey into Day:
    Issues for Therapists, Counselors,
    Clergy and Carers   44
7   Awakening Meaning: The Spiritual
    Dimension of Healing   49

Part Three
AIDS AND COMMUNITY GROWTH

8	The Issue of Screening and the Educational Challenge	59
9	Transformation: Personal and Collective	64
10	Relationships: Integrating Sexuality and Spirituality	71

Part Four
PSYCHOTHERAPY, COUNSELING AND PASTORAL CARE: ACTIVITIES AND EXERCISES

11	Relaxation, Visualization, Meditation and Reflections for Discussion	81
	'Ecce Homo!': Behold the Man!—88. Homosexuality and the 'Natural Law'—91. Oppression, Stigma and the Killing Process—94. Denial: Its Many Faces—99. Repression and Morality—101. Sexuality and the Search for Transcendence—104. SOMA: Society Of Marvellous Acceptance—107. Religious Communities: Models and Structures—110.	
12	Spiritual Exercises with Archetypal Images and Symbols	114
	Light and Darkness—115. Water—117. Bread and Wine—122. Incense: Celebrating and Remembering—126. Anointing with Oil, Healing Touch and Washing—129. The Use of Icons—133.	

POSTSCRIPT	A Dream of Gerontius	138
APPENDIX	Presenting Patients: What to Look for and How	141
BIBLIOGRAPHY		146
INDEX OF TOPICS		149

PREFACE

One of the extraordinary triumphs of the human spirit is the ability to transcend tragedy and find intimations of a finer destiny in contending with the fear and depression that can haunt our human condition.

Peter Todd has contemplated the fearful and depressing facts of the HIV epidemic that first came to the notice of medical science ten years ago. Now, in this book, he examines the voluminous literature of clinical medicine and its allied social sciences and seeks to utilize those insights in his own practice of psychotherapy. Basing his practice on that solid and growing knowledge base, Peter worked for several years as psychologist-therapist with people who were coping with the alarm and perplexity of finding themselves infected with the human immune virus. From that cumulative experience Peter developed a therapy which promotes well-being and serenity in the face of obsessive anxiety and dread about the outcome of infection. This book tells of the way that those affected by HIV or AIDS can surmount their fears and win serenity even in the face of pain and loss and death. Remarkably this is a book about hope and affection and courage; it celebrates the human condition through an odyssey of discovery—a realisation of the divine potential of being human. The book took me on an exciting journey and I pressed on rapidly to form an overall understanding of this philosophical approach to healing.

The first section presents an intriguing perspective on psychosomatic medicine, psychoneuroimmunology and especially their application to immune-deficiency conditions. Chapter one introduces the sustaining themes. The second chapter's engaging account of the work of Freud and its subsequent implementation in psychosomatic medicine and psychotherapy engrossed me. The excursion into Popperian logic and its tolerance for inquiry, until falsification, diverts briefly before engaging with Jung and Frankl, whose influence on Todd's therapeutic work becomes more and more apparent. Chapter three presents a cameo-history of the development of psychoneuroimmunology that is accessible to the lay-reader. The linking of the psychosocial dimensions of lived experience to health and illness argues persuasively for the relevance of the therapies put forward in later chapters.

In Part Two we move on to consider the applications of these philosophical insights to contemporary conditions, to current ills. The study reported in chapter four points to radical changes in the way we should treat people whose health is jeopardized by immune-suppression; Todd's study of AIDS and AIDS-related conditions clearly has implications for cancer treatments and, probably, for dealing with a wide range of immune-related diseases. This chapter sets out the case for acceptance (in this case of homosexual identity) and argues powerfully for the therapeutic value of accepting one's own sexual integrity and being. It points further to the importance of knowing and accepting ourselves and our human condition (general as well as specific to place and time).

Then begins Todd's account of therapies which have proved effective in promoting healing and serenity. These are directed to modifying the psychological factors which can diminish immunity imperiled by HIV or AIDS. Much of this draws upon and explains the dynamics of group psychotherapy. Todd does not dodge the hard questions. Later chapters take this further and tell of troubling issues confronting counselors as well as clients, offering practical and creative strategies. Depression, aggression transference, countertransference, futility, suicide are to be dealt with. Exhaustion and burn-out are to be avoided. Todd describes strategies for all these purposes. The spiritual dimensions of discovering the meaning in one's living come to the fore by the end of this section; the promised pilgrimage into healing becomes clear.

Part Three is challenging and comforting. I am not personally convinced that everyone who thinks themselves at risk should be tested for HIV. But the points Todd makes do persuade me that this is, for most people, a sound initiative. The decision not to be tested does reflect fear and defensiveness, which emanates from the belief that nothing can be done to affect the outcome. The research papers cited here may be the stance of David against the grim Goliath of the mass of clinical opinion. The conventional wisdom gives little support at the individual level for the desirability of finding out one's HIV status. But, Todd's approach is about looking fear in the face and, by knowing, overcoming it.

People, including those who profess no religion, look to religion for possible answers to questions of well-being, or illness, or death. In a western context this usually means that Christian religions are in the forefront of this questioning, although our secularism and our religious pluralism imply that responses can come from many different religious and spiritual spheres. AIDS confronts organized religions and requires inspired responses. Peter Todd takes us to his world view and that may be different from our own. This book is about one intensely personal pilgrimage, one that can be widely but not universally shared.

The book examines issues that all counselors and psychotherapists, including the most pragmatic and materialist, must consider—the underlying psychological factors of simple human responsibility. This is good psychology, good sociology and good materialist logic.

In the final section Todd shows his highly developed and spiritually informed psychotherapy. This is embedded in a deeply religious culture. The symbolism is widely shared, in Jungian terms much is universal, and the imagery resonates with several world religions, particularly Todd's early Catholicism. This is the stuff of dreams and hopes; it is a personal vision and one inspiring a great following. Todd writes of a movement into spirituality, but ours is a very secular society and this last section will surprise, even alarm, some readers.

The therapeutic exercises (which remind me of the concept of Ignatius' spiritual exercises) are soundly based in the more spiritual culture of Christianity. For other cultures, other rituals are efficacious. The intentions and meanings of these exercises are universal, the ways of representing them are, of necessity, culturally bound.

Peter Todd pleads persuasively for an AIDS outreach, for models of compassionate community which will respect the locus of of control in the individual and build loving awareness of others. The postscript which shares the final pilgrimage and dream, while the friend 'Gerontius' dies, is profoundly moving.

The book is a healing catharsis. Its readership lies with all those people affected by, working with, or interested in the issue of AIDS. It should be read in universities, especially in those faculties concerned with education and training for counseling, therapy and a holistic approach to medicine.

Ann Daniel
Associate Professor and Head of Sociology
University of New South Wales

INTRODUCTION
The Miracle of Wholeness

The theme of this book is that the miracles of healing and of wholeness begin with persons. Health means a unity or integration of body, mind and spirit. Mounting research evidence now suggests that diseases such as cancer, autoimmune disorders and infections reflect personality and emotional factors as well as biological ones. Moreover, frustration or blockage of personal growth and the search for meaning appear to contribute to disease-proneness.

Our approach to patients should therefore address the full biopsychosocial reality of the human condition. In other words, illnesses are processes reflecting the total system of individuals and their environment—ecology in the broadest sense. One problem with the traditional medical model is that it tends to neglect the psychological and spiritual dimensions of health and disease.

Overcoming AIDS will, in my opinion, require a revolution in scientific understanding and caring for patients. The chapters which follow attempt to explain why. They may also be read as steps in a pilgrimage to healing, recovery and personal growth, as well as a guide to the prevention of illness in at-risk or HIV-infected persons.

The presence of HIV/AIDS, represents an ultimate challenge, not only to the health-care systems, but also to society and to the churches. For, in the pastoral and sacramental care of HIV antibody positive persons and their partners and families lies a unique opportunity for compassionate outreach, reconciliation and healing.

As the chapters that follow will suggest, people living with AIDS, all too often carry within themselves the deep wounds of social oppression, homophobia and stigmatization, all of which renders many of them more susceptible to HIV, once infected. The church, as an institution, has, however unwittingly, often contributed to this wounding insofar as it has tended to buttress homophobic and judgemental attitudes in society.

As a result, may people now living with HIV/AIDS remain alienated; cut off from the vast spiritual treasures of sacrament, liturgy and means of grace, forgiveness, wholeness and healing. However, such persons might well represent one of the most obvious and poignant manifestations of the suffering face of Jesus Christ himself.

The content of this book reflects my indebtedness to many persons. First, I wish to thank Associate Professor Wendy Walker of the Department of Behavioural Sciences in Medicine, Sydney University, for a quarter-century of inspiration and encouragement. Second, I owe much to Associate Professor Christopher Magarey of the Department of Surgery, the St George Hospital, Sydney, for several years of very fruitful collaboration in research into psychological aspects of breast cancer and for his vision into emotional and spiritual dimensions of healing. Finally, I want to thank the members of the Biopsychosocial AIDS Project, University of California, San Francisco, for their generous advice in particular, Professor George Solomon and my colleagues, including Tim Keogh, for valuable friendship and support.

This book is written primarily for health professionals clergy, educators and carers—all those who work with HIV-infected persons. The vast research in psychosomatic medicine and from the emerging field of psychoneuroimmunology has vital implications for therapies aiming to prevent illness in individuals exposed to HIV, that is, for the goal of secondary prevention. However, the book is dedicated to my patients, many of whom have been models of courage and heroism.

PART ONE

THE ASCENT OF HOLISM

CHAPTER ONE
Revolutions in Understanding and Caring

The 'Germ Theory'

For almost 150 years, the 'Germ Theory', according to which diseases are caused by external agents invading hosts, has dominated western medicine. This theory has revolutionized the diagnosis and treatment of many diseases which had previously either decimated populations or resulted in countless premature deaths.

Related discoveries of antisepsis, vaccination and antibiotics, as well as anaesthesia, x-rays, refined surgical techniques and chemical therapies, raised the optimistic hope that humanity stood on the threshold of conquering all disease. Perhaps too the secret wish for immortality, embodied in John Donne's sixteenth century sonnet, 'Death Be Not Proud,' was about to be fulfilled!

Nemesis

However, the 'Germ Theory' or, more generally, the medical model, rested upon a rather dubious assumption. This was the belief that knowledge of the causal role of biological factors alone was sufficient to explain the occurrence of disease.

The early triumphs of the medical model resulted in much power, privilege and status being given to the medical profession. Linked with this was a growing tendency to view patients as purely passive recipients of medical services. Thus, people's personal power and ability to accept responsibility for their own health and healing were all too frequently denied or minimized.

Many individual doctors are caring, idealistic persons. However, an almost magical reliance upon technology has tended to create alienation or distance between healers and patients, instead of shared responsibility and dialogue. Communication skills and empathy have been neglected and instead of a concern for whole persons, it has become safer and easier to focus only upon, 'the malignant breast lump in bed X' or 'the cardiac arrest in room Y'. Yet extensive research evidence suggests that perceived personal power or control over health on the part of the patient, and the expression of negative emotions such as hostility, predict a better prognosis in diseases such as cancer. Being a 'bad' patient tends to predict a better chance of recovery!

In summary, patients often tend to be de-personalized, made into 'objects' to be treated with mechanical procedures, as though healing occurred only in isolated organ systems or body parts. The psychological and spiritual dimensions of healing are often perceived as irrelevant and therefore ignored.

The 'nemesis of medicine', described brilliantly by Ivan Illich, mirrors both unresolved paradoxes and factual questions associated with the medical model and the 'desacralization of science', as described by Abraham Maslow in his book *The Psychology of Science*. In banishing the psyche, the soul, from the sanctuaries of respectable scientific enquiry and treatment, we have created idols fashioned from narrow concepts of science (scientism) and the products of technology, with resulting gaps in understanding and caring for patients.

Failure to perceive these limitations is due to our Western prejudice and arrogance which leads to a neglect of healing practices used in other cultures for centuries. It is as though we had nothing to learn!

Crisis

In reality, scientific understanding of diseases such as cancer, mental illness, alcoholism and now AIDS is still very far from being complete. Moreover, the belief that comprehensive explanation of these disorders will eventually be achieved within the confines of the medical model appears to be illusory. The factual basis of this claim will be outlined in subsequent chapters.

Limitations in caring and treatment clearly reflect these gaps in scientific knowledge. In fact, the existence of so many outstanding puzzles, which seem to defy solution when approached within the medical model, suggests the diagnosis of an acute identity crisis in medicine. An appropriate remedy will require a radical dissection of the anatomy of the medical model and a thorough grasp of its limitations.

Paradoxes

Thomas Kuhn in his book *The Structure of Scientific Revolutions* has analyzed the factors which generate crises for theories and models. Kuhn discusses also how such crises have set the stage for revolutions in such fields as astronomy, chemistry and biology.

These scientific revolutions had key elements in common. The elements included a combination of unresolved problems, paradoxes or anomalies, *the persistence of which suggested that particular theories had exhausted their usefulness as explanatory tools*. The emergence of vital facts, not anticipated or adequately explained within the theory, resulted in crises and ultimately, in ingenious new theories. Such theories, made up of new analogies, metaphors, symbolic generalizations or empirical laws, often implied a radical inversion of world-view!

For example, the Copernican Theory that the earth revolved around the sun and not vice-versa, resulted in the abandonment of the older Ptolemaic concept which had dominated astronomy for more than a thousand years. However, the political and social implications were extraordinary, for Ptolemy's theory had become enshrined as a dogma in Christian theology. The idea that the earth and therefore the human race was the centre of the universe seemed consistent with the biblical doctrine of creation. Copernicus' theory was therefore threatening to theologians of the day—to such an extent that his disciple, Bruno, was burned at the stake for heresy for refusing to abandon the new view.

Revolutions of similar magnitude are associated with the names of Charles Darwin in biology, for proposing the theory of evolution by the natural selection of chance variations, and Sigmund Freud, who upset rationalist concepts by demonstrating the unconscious motivation of much human behaviour, including symptoms of disorders such as conversion hysteria which had been considered neurological illnesses.

Anomalies, paradoxes and problems which persist and seem unlikely to be solved within the framework of the medical model, have created a crisis and the need for a revolution in medicine. It is time to consider these questions and puzzles in more detail, to understand why.

A Revolution in Medicine

What are the unresolved puzzles and paradoxes? Consider cancer. Lung cancer is not randomly distributed in the smoking population, even allowing for quantity of smoking and its duration. Psychological factors appear to be significant. The research of Kissen and others, reported in his paper 'Psychosocial Factors, Personality and Lung Cancer in Men Aged Between 55 and 64,' indicates that such factors as the inability to express emotions ('diminished outlets for emotional discharge') and the use of defense mechanisms such as denial and repression contribute significantly to susceptibility.

Extensive research, including that of Bahnson, Greer, Magarey and Todd (papers listed in the Bibliography) suggests that the onset and course of malignancy are strongly influenced by emotional factors. These include suppressed negative emotions, especially anger, loss of significant relationships, depression, giving-up and the use of repression and denial as defences against threat. The pioneering work of these investigators, as well as the contributions of Engel, Schmale, Levy and many others discussed later, has revealed a remarkably consistent pattern of psychological factors predicting either the onset or progression of cancer, irrespective of bodily site.

Even more extraordinary, however, are the converging or parallel results of studies of personality, stress and emotional factors predicting the onset and courses of other immune-related disorders such as rheumatoid arthritis and infections such as herpes simplex and infectious mononucleosis. Solomon, another pioneer in psychoneuroimmunology (see chapter three), has coined the suggestive term, 'immunosuppression-prone personality pattern,' to denote this consistency of relevant psychological factors.

More recently, my own research on the possible role of psychological factors in the development of T-cell immune defects and symptoms of the 'AIDS-Related Complex' (ARC), has provided significant data consistent with this notion. Such data, reported briefly in chapter four, also highlight the likely relevance of psychological interventions, such as group psychotherapy, counseling and visualization as means of possibly influencing immunity and illness in HIV infection. Magarey and others have reported similar work relevant to cancer and this is summarized later.

It is known that personality, stress and lifestyle factors increase the risk of heart disease (for example, the so-called Type-A Personality). Alcoholism, defined as a disease by the World Health Organization, is notoriously unresponsive to medical approaches. The most powerful and effective treatment, provided by Alcoholics Anonymous, is in fact a *spiritual* program.

In summary, the significance of these kinds of facts is that the medical model does not and probably cannot account for the individual variations in the onset and course of many major life-threatening illnesses. It neither allows for comprehensive explanation, nor does it provide a basis for modifying significant, causally-relevant, non-biological factors.

Such anomalies and unresolvable problems are the stuff of which scientific revolutions are made. The medical model now needs to be replaced with one which permits more adequate explanation and caring. Engel, a pioneer in psychosomatic research, describes his perception of 'the need for a new medical model,' and the pertinence of a 'biopsychosocial' approach in two seminal papers, written towards the end of the 1970s. Such a 'holistic' or 'multi-factorial' model now seems likely to provide a better fit to the currently available facts.

CHAPTER TWO

The Origins of Holism and Psychosomatics

In the history of ideas, the notion that the psyche somehow influences disease is not new. For example, the ancient Greek physician Galen believed that a connection existed between 'melancholia' (depression) and malignancy, specifically breast cancer.

Modern medicine, however, has adopted a mechanistic view of human beings and a materialist concept of illness, reflecting, among other factors, the influence of Newtonian physics. In a clockwork universe, described by elegant equations, the psyche is reduced to brain states—the subtle interplay of nerve-impulses and chemical messengers. Indeed, until the rise of the psychosomatic approach, the mind was exorcised from the domain of proper medical-scientific enquiry. Patients with spiritual concerns were quietly referred to theologians.

The Freudian Revolution

Sigmund Freud, the father of psychoanalysis, is perhaps best known for his theory of the unconscious motives and conflicts behind neurotic symptoms, as well as dreams and errors. His discoveries are described best in his own literary style in books such as *The Interpretation of Dreams* and *The Psychopathology of Everyday Life*. Freud began his brilliant career, however, as a neurologist, making important contributions to the development of anaesthesia (he studied and used cocaine) and to the understanding of disorders which had puzzled his medical colleagues. His case studies of conversion hysteria, carried out with Joseph Breuer, revealed that hysterical paralysis and blindness, previously thought to be organic, neurological disorders, were in fact caused by repressed, unconscious conflicts about sexuality and aggression. These discoveries were made using hypnosis and later dream interpretation and free-association, which laid the foundations of psychoanalysis.

However, the main historical significance of Freud's early work for the rise of psychosomatic medicine was that of revealing vital gaps in concepts of diseases which were considered to be purely organic or neurological in origin. His theory of a *dynamic unconscious level of motivation* really paved the way for later psychosomatic concepts of illness.

For example, Bahnson, a pioneer in work with cancer patients, wrote (1970): 'In cancer patients, the phenomenological (subjective) state of depression (repressed rage) is denied or repressed and discharged instead somatically within the organism.' Repressed emotional conflicts, especially about loss of significant persons, depression and anger were, according to Bahnson, translated into bodily illness, in this case, cancer. How this might happen was still, at this time, largely a matter of speculation. Answers would come later from the emerging science of psychoneuroimmunology, discussed in the next chapter under the heading of 'biological mechanisms'.

The Context of Discovery

The revolution begun by Freud was mirrored in the clinical observations of persons trained in or familiar with psychoanalysis in patients with diverse somatic disorders. These illnesses included cancer and infections. One of the most influential early clinicians was Alexander, author of *Psychosomatic Medicine*, published in 1950. Alexander related psychological factors to seven disease entities including peptic ulcer, ulcerative colitis, hyperthyroidism, rheumatoid arthritis and bronchial asthma. Other pioneers included Engel, Grinker and Nemiah, as well as Kissen who made significant contributions to psychosomatic concepts of cancer.

Evaluating much of the early, largely clinical work in psychosomatic medicine is facilitated by a useful distinction made by Philosopher Karl Popper in his book *The Logic of Scientific Discovery*. This is the distinction between what Popper refers to as the 'context of discovery' and that of 'justification'.

The 'context of discovery' is simply the lived-through stream of experience in which scientists make connections between previously unrelated events, for example, psychological and biological or clinical ones. This is the matrix or source of inspiration and theories about what goes with what. However, observations made in this (discovery) context are not a sufficient basis for testing the scientific 'truth' value of one's ideas or hypotheses. Too many possibilities for error and self-deception exist!

The testing or verification of hypotheses requires a further step which takes place in what Popper calls the 'context of justification'. In this context, experiments or controlled empirical enquiries, consisting of systematic observations, the use of control groups and the apparatus of inferential statistics, permit calculation of the probability that a given hypothesis is true in comparison with others. A given set of findings that could have occurred by chance alone at less than an agreed level (say, five times in one hundred) is said to be 'significant'. If such a significance level is achieved, the hypothesis is accepted as verified, although always open to subsequent falsification in the light of new evidence.

The logic and structure of such scientific investigations are complex and beyond the scope of this book. However, these methods are described in many sources, including the texts by Popper and Nagel listed in the Bibliography.

The essential point of this section and the reason for the brief digression into scientific methodology, is that *much early work in psychosomatic medicine really belonged in the 'context of discovery'*. The findings were not yet verified scientific fact, but rather, a source of ingenious ideas or hypotheses for systematic study. Is this distinction pedantic or purely academic and why is it important?

It is not, I believe, pedantic! For instance, these days some proponents of so-called 'holistic' approaches to cancer and AIDS are tempted to make extravagant claims about alleged links between such things as nutrition, lifestyles, vitamin C and meditation on the one hand and immune status or the course of illness on the other. All too often such claims are not based upon properly conducted scientific studies or subjected to rigorous hypothesis-testing. The result is that the holistic model itself is brought into disrepute and patients may be encouraged to embrace treatments which may have no value at all. One eminent professor I know keeps a file labelled 'Cancer Quackery' into which reports about contentious or spurious 'therapies' are placed regularly!

The Resurrection of Meaning

The possible relevance of the spiritual dimension of meaning, commitment and purpose to survival and disease-proneness received much of its early impetus from the work of Viennese psychiatrist Viktor Frankl who was interned in Auschwitz. Frankl confronted the question of what factors characterized survivors in such extreme situations as the Nazi concentration camps. He observed that persons who experienced a sense of meaning in life, whether commitment to a partner, love for a community, unfinished tasks or belief in a personal God, seemed far more likely to survive. Those who perceived life as meaningless or succumbed to hopelessness, were more likely, in his view, to die of immune-related illnesses (infections) or to commit suicide.

Many other clinicians and social scientists have contributed to this resurrection of the spiritual dimension and its possible role in survival and healing. Carl Jung, a contemporary of Freud, greatly extended the notion of the unconscious to include spiritual factors. The work of Erich Fromm and Abraham Maslow as leaders of the humanistic movement in psychology will be referred to later. However, these writers seemed to share the belief that spirituality was somehow related to healing and growth. 'Self-actualization' meant a move away from self-centredness towards Other- or God-centredness. Growth implied coming to perceive oneself as part of a larger social-cultural-spiritual whole and then contributing to that whole.

Kobasa's research work, reported in such papers as 'Stressful Life Events, Personality and Health: An Enquiry into Hardiness,' has explored the relevance of meaning to disease-proneness and is generally supportive of the formulations of Jung, Maslow, Fromm and others.

Holism Defined

This chapter has summarized briefly the emergence of factors other than purely biological ones which may be causally-relevant to disease. It has traced the origins of what is now called a 'biopsychosocial' or 'holistic' model of illness.

The primary assumption of this model is that knowledge of biological or organic factors *alone* is not sufficient for comprehensive scientific explanation or as a basis for treatment or caring. Further, comprehensive explanation will entail obtaining information about the psychological, social and spiritual factors influencing susceptibility to agents such as viruses and carcinogens (cancer-inducing products, e.g. toxic chemicals). If we all swim in a sea of carcinogens, then the question as to why some people are more vulnerable to such agents is likely to be answered to a significant extent by an understanding of the role of psychological factors. The same issue applies to HIV infection.

Holism, then, encompasses scientific evidence about *all* of the measurable, causally-significant factors, including psychological, social and spiritual ones. In the next chapter, I explore in more depth some of the fascinating links already shown by research to exist between personality, stress, emotions, immunity and disease. This subject matter forms a vital part of the content of a relatively new science called 'psychoneuroimmunology'.

This is an exciting field of scientific enquiry because it seems to be opening up novel pathways to the enhanced understanding and effective treatment of persons with life-threatening diseases, such as cancer and AIDS. The research data also have vital implications for the prevention of illness in HIV antibody positive persons, with early psychosocial interventions.

CHAPTER THREE

Psychoneuroimmunology: Emotions, Immunity and Disease

Psychoneuroimmunology is a lusty new science. It explores links between psychological factors and the onset and course of diseases which reflect breakdown of the immune system. These diseases include cancer, autoimmune disorders such as rheumatoid arthritis and infections such as herpes simplex and infectious mononucleosis. More recently, the powerful conceptual tools of this science have been used to help generate an enhanced understanding of AIDS.

Crucial to this domain of scientific enquiry is the detailed study of the biological mechanisms or pathways whereby personality, stress and emotional factors might be translated into disease. These will be discussed later in this chapter.

Sometimes, the term 'psychoimmunology' is substituted for the longer word 'psychoneuroimmunology'. However, this usage tends to result in overlooking the complexity and richness of certain biological pathways, especially the role of neurotransmitters ('chemical messengers') and hormones in the communication network which exists between the brain and the immune system. Before we consider the relevance of this field to the understanding of such diseases as cancer and AIDS, it would be helpful to summarize briefly some of the work in psychosomatic medicine which promoted the rise of psychoneuroimmunology.

The Specificity Hypothesis

The pioneering work in psychosomatic medicine was carried out by such eminent clinicians and research workers as Alexander, Nemiah, Grinker, Bahnson, Kissen and Engel, to name just a few. All, in a sense, stood on the shoulders of Freud and other psychoanalytic theorists, being influenced by such concepts as 'repression of emotions', 'inward-turning anger or rage', and the 'somatization of unconscious conflicts'. According to these workers, organ systems become diseased because of the 'damming-up' of negative feelings, such as anger, or the use of defense mechanisms such as denial and repression.

Implicit in the work was the notion that it not stress per se that is pathogenic, but rather the person's appraisal of and defense against threat. Thus, ineffective or failing coping or defense mechanisms were thought to be mirrored at a biological level, although details of how were to be an issue for later more sophisticated research into the physiological correlates of emotions and defensive failure.

One early notion was the so-called 'specificity hypothesis': specific personality factors or unconscious conflicts were thought to be causally relevant to particular diseases or even to 'symbolically-significant' organs such as the breast. A related, optimistic belief was that certain variations of psychoanalytic therapy might result in a cure or recovery from illnesses such as bronchial asthma or rheumatoid arthritis.

Even Bahnson, writing in the early 1970s, expressed the view that progress with cancer might depend upon 'resolving core psychodynamic conflicts,' especially those concerning loss of significant persons, depression and the repression of negative emotions such as anger or rage. Later work has supported the relevance of these sorts of factors to immune-related diseases *generally*, not just to cancer.

More sophisticated research work in the last decade has resulted in the demise of the 'specificity hypothesis'. It has been replaced by a more plausible, scientifically-supported concept, highlighting *common factors* in the onset and outcome of many diseases which reflect dysfunction or breakdown of the immune system.

The Immunosuppression-Prone Personality Pattern

Recent work in psychoneuroimmunology has led to a remarkable discovery, germane to the dominant theme of this book. This is the emergence of the concept referred to by Solomon as 'the immunosuppression-prone personality pattern'. This is a pattern of psychological factors relevant to the onset and progression of almost all of the major immune-related diseases so far studied by researchers in the field of psychoneuroimmunology. Technical details are provided in Solomon's papers, listed in the Bibliography. However, I shall list the most significant factors:

- Defense mechanisms used to ward off stress and threat, such as denial and repression.

- The effectiveness of these defense or coping mechanisms in warding off noxious emotions such as anxiety. Failure of defenses seems to be mirrored in changes in the biological mechanisms by which emotional factors influence disease.

- Ego-strength or resiliency, that is, a person's capacity for flexible adaptation to change or stress. Jemmott and Locke, whose papers are listed in the Bibliography, report data on the relevance of this factor.

- Object-loss, that is, loss of significant persons through death or separation, and so-called 'symbolic losses', for example, of career, power, body-image. Bartrop, an Australian physician, was the first in the world to demonstrate immune-suppression after bereavement and his findings were confirmed by Schleifer.

- Depression, thought to be symptomatic of 'inward-turning anger' and usually also a component or stage of grieving.

- Hopelessness or giving-up, as shown for example, in the work of Schmale and others on cervical cancer in women.

- Emotional control or expressiveness in regard to negative emotions such as anger, predictive of breast cancer prognosis in the work of Greer and his colleagues.

- Perceived locus of control over life events or health status. People may believe that what happens to their health is due to external factors such as fate or chance or the influence of powerful others or that health depends upon their own efforts. An internal locus of control or a sense of personal power over one's health seems to predict a better prognosis in a number of conditions, including, possibly, HIV infection.

- Social support or alienation.

- Integration of sexual identity (shown by my own work, reported in chapter four, to be a powerful predictor of immune status).

- The spiritual dimension of meaning and commitment, the relevance of which has already been discussed.

Key papers reporting studies of the relevance of all of these factors to immunity and disease include those by Bahnson, Crisp, Greer, Jemmott, Levy, Kobasa, Schmale, Solomon, Magarey and Todd and are included in the Bibliography.

Beyond Correlations

A major weakness in many early studies in psychosomatic medicine was the reporting of correlations, sometimes with implied causal significance. However, correlations between psychological factors and disease, no matter how statistically significant, do not *necessarily* allow causal inferences to be made.

Several reasons exist for this. Firstly, measures of certain personality and emotional factors might themselves reflect the influence of disease or knowledge of diagnosis. Secondly, apparent correlations may be due to the effects of additional or spurious factors. For example, simply demonstrating a correlation between, say, depression and cancer incidence does not in itself suffice to establish a causal connection. To make this inference, one must first control for the known relationship between both cancer and depression and *age*. This is because both cancer and depression are more common with increasing age. An excellent review of these sorts of issues is provided by Fox in his paper 'Psychosocial Factors in the Immune System in Human Cancer,' listed in the Bibliography.

An even more substantial problem with simple correlational studies is the absence of data concerning *how* personality, stress or emotional factors might influence disease. This is the critical issue of knowing the biological mechanisms or pathways by which such factors could be translated into pathophysiological changes, in other words, into symptoms of diseases, such as cancer or AIDS.

Biological Mechanisms

Current research in psychoneuroimmunology is exploring the question of how measured psychological factors might influence disease. This means assessing links between these factors and changes in key components of the immune system as well as in neurotransmitters and hormones which assist in the translation of emotional factors into immune changes. Vital components of cellular immunity under study include T-cells (produced by the thymus gland) and natural killer cells, known to be essential in the surveillance and destruction of alien or abnormal cells, such as cancer cells and virus-infected cells.

Significant relationships have already been found between such stressors as bereavement, life-change stress, emotions such as suppressed anger and depression, defences such as denial and changes in components of cellular immunity. Bartrop's work on immuno-suppression (reduction in T-lymphocytes) following bereavement has been referred to already. Other pertinent papers, concerning the influence of psychological factors on T-cells, natural killer cell activity and other immune variables, include those by Schleifer, Jemmott, Levy, Locke, Greer, Todd and many others. These papers are listed in the Bibliography and several are included in Ader's volume entitled, *Psychoneuroimmunology* which is a comprehensive, though technical review of work prior to 1981.

With regard to other mechanisms, much work has also been done on the role of hormones, neurotransmitters and recently, mast-cells, at the interface of the central nervous and immune systems. Elaborate feedback loops involving thymic hormones (e.g. thymosin alpha one), important in the development and differentiation of T-cells and cortisol, known to be immunosuppressive, have already been mapped out.

Receptors for neurotransmitters have been discovered on T-lymphocytes, and mast-cells appear to 'translate' nerve impulses into chemical signals read by thymic and splenic lymphocytes. In short, an exquisite communications network exists between the brain and the immune system. This provides the beginnings of a biological basis for the impact of psychological factors upon immune-related illnesses such as cancer and AIDS, albeit in a highly simplistic form, which leaves a very complex mystery to be explored.

However, much work remains to be done before these complex pathways are understood fully. This is clearly the future challenge of research in the field of psychoneuroimmunology.

Practical Implications

A vital dimension of healing appears to be opening up because of the recent developments in psychoneuroimmunology. Therapies, designed to modify relevant psychological factors, should result in changes in both immunity and disease. Part Two of this book focuses largely upon the elaboration of such practical implications. However, first, the next chapter describes research relevant to the rise of a holistic or multifactorial model of AIDS.

PART TWO
RAISING CONSCIOUSNESS

CHAPTER FOUR

A Holistic or Biopsychosocial Model of AIDS

Causality: Necessary and Sufficient Conditions

Comprehensive scientific understanding of AIDS will entail obtaining knowledge of psychological factors influencing host susceptibility, disease onset and outcome, once infection with the human immunodeficiency virus (HIV) has occurred. In terms of a multifactorial or holistic model of illness, exposure to HIV can be considered a *necessary* condition for the development of clinical illness. However, the *sufficient* conditions will include psychological and social factors.

Scientific evidence concerning the relevance of such factors to immune suppression and illness onset and outcome in HIV infection is also vital as a foundation for psychosocial interventions aiming to prevent illness onset as well as to enhance survival time. The overall aim of the study reported briefly in this chapter was to explore links between personality, stress and emotional factors on the one hand and the development of defects in T-cell immunity and the onset of clinical symptoms on the other.

Subjects and Methods

The subjects consisted of 175 of the almost 1,000 homosexual or bisexual men enrolled in the Sydney AIDS Project between February 1984 and January 1985. Subjects were enrolled by medical practitioners after obtaining informed consent. The 175 subjects assessed in the psychosocial part of the study were similar to those in the overall project, with respect to demographic factors such as age, socio-economic status and education. Details of demography, epidemiological, clinical and laboratory investigations are described in the AIDS issue of the *Medical Journal of Australia*, October 1984.

In the psychoneuroimmunological component of the study, subjects were given standardized psychological scales of known reliability to measure relevant factors. Details of these instruments are reported elsewhere (Todd and others, 1987 and 1988, listed in the Bibliography). The following psychological factors were assessed: (a) defense mechanisms, denial and repression; (b) ego-strength (resiliency); (c) depression; (d) hopelessness; (e) emotional control/expressiveness; (f) object-loss (death or separation in the last three years); (g) perceived control (personal power) over health status; (h) social support; (i) integration (acceptance) of gay identity.

Laboratory tests included those determining antibody status to HIV and measures of T-cell subsets, including T4 and T8 numbers, from which the 'helper/suppressor ratio' could be calculated. Again, technical details are reported in the October 1984 issue of the *Medical Journal of Australia* and in Todd's 1987 and 1988 papers, listed in the Bibliography.

Results

The significance of links between measured psychological factors, the development of defects in T-cell immunity and the onset of symptoms of the so-called 'AIDS-Related

Complex' (ARC), was tested using multivariate statistical techniques. These methods, called discriminant function and logistic regression analyses are mathematical tools for evaluating the influence of multiple factors in predicting an outcome or criterion, such as whether or not people develop T-cell immune defects or experience the onset of symptoms. Technical details of these methods are beyond the scope of this book and are provided in the original papers (Todd, 1987, 1988) and in the books by Cooley & Lohnes and Klecka (see Bibliography).

Psychological Factors Discriminating T-cell Immune Defects

The factors significant in discriminating the presence or absence of defects in T-cell immunity in HIV antibody positive (infected) subjects were: (a) suppression of depression; (b) acceptance of gay identity; (c) the use of denial and repression as defences; (d) explosive expression of anger in frustrating situations; (e) termination (loss) of a relationship with one's partner in the last three years. Suppression of depression, explosive expression of anger and termination of a relationship were associated with a *much greater likelihood of developing a defect in T-cell immunity*, once infected with HIV. Acceptance of gay-identity and the effective use of denial and repression as defences were associated with a *much lesser likelihood of developing T-cell immune defects*. The implications, of these findings for therapeutic interventions are discussed below.

Psychological Factors Discriminating ARC and Healthy Status

The factors significant in predicting which subjects would be diagnosed with AIDS-Related Complex (ARC) or retain healthy, asymptomatic status, were: (a) suppression of anger; (b) manifest (expressed) anxiety; (c) death of partner from any cause in the last three years; (d) suppression/control of depression and (e) self-reported symptoms of depression. The factors of internalized stigma (homophobia), inward-turning anger, termination of relationship with partner and perceived locus of control over health, classified subjects in the predicted direction, but fell short of statistical significance.

Of these factors, suppression of anger, death of partner and self-reported depressive symptoms were associated with *a much greater likelihood of a diagnosis of ARC*. The manifest expression of anxiety and suppression/control of depressed feelings were associated with *a much lesser likelihood of ARC diagnosis and with the maintenance of healthy, asymptomatic status*.

Significance Levels and Individual Variation

Both of the above analyses yielded results significant at beyond the 0.0001 level of probability. In other words, the results could have occurred *by chance alone less than one time in ten thousand*, a highly statistically significant outcome. Moreover, significant psychological factors accounted for 54.6 per cent of the individual variation in developing defects in T-cell immunity among seropositive subjects. Significant psychological factors also accounted for 37.2 per cent of the individual variation in whether or not subjects received a diagnosis of ARC, as opposed to retaining healthy, asymptomatic status.

In simple terms, measured psychological factors accounted for more than half of what happened with respect to the development of T-cell immune defects and for more than one-third of the outcome with respect to the onset of symptoms of AIDS-Related Complex (ARC).

Discussion

The overall results are quite consistent with published data as well as supportive of hypotheses about links between excessive control (suppression) of negative emotions and the onset and course of other immune-related diseases. However, it is quite possible that some complex (non-linear) relationships exist. For example, both extreme over-control (suppression) and excessive expression of anger or rage might be immunosuppressive. Thus, assertiveness and the constructive channeling or appropriate expression of such emotions might be both adaptive and more likely to be linked with intact immunity and health. The destructive acting-out of previously repressed rage, on the other hand, would be maladaptive socially and associated with immune suppression.

Jemmott (1984) has reported such a non-linear relationship between life-change stress and antibody response. The issue of the existence of such complex relationships, however, remains to be resolved through future research, using sophisticated statistical techniques.

The finding of a significant link between *acceptance of gay identity and a lesser likelihood of developing T-cell immune defects* is important and has not, to the author's knowledge, been reported previously. It has implications for therapy and is significant because traditionally many health professionals have regarded homosexuality itself as a symptom of maladjustment or 'psychopathology'. The work of Vivienne Cass and others on homosexual identity formation has contributed to a gradual change in this view. Judd Marmor, in his *Homosexual Behaviour: A Modern Reappraisal*, provides a detailed review of the need, on clinical grounds, to change negative attitudes, aside from the fact that the homosexual condition or orientation itself is no longer regarded as a personality disorder which either requires treatment or is in any case susceptible to change in the majority of cases.

Since homosexuality, as an orientation and an affectional

preference, as well as a dimension of personal identity, is now known to be irreversibly formed early in life, by about the age of four to six years, it is likely that *accepting* this vital part of the self would minimize clinical psychopathology and self-destructive behaviour patterns, through the person's life-cycle. Such acceptance of homosexual identity would also open up a capacity for loving and those channels of emotional expression, now known to be predictive of the susceptibility to and progression of cancer, revealed in the above mentioned studies of Kissen, Greer and others. Acceptance, not repression, would facilitate *sublimation*, for example, in the religious life, in which sacrificial renunciation might be a meaningful option or way of coping.

The association of repression and denial with a lesser likelihood of a T-cell immune-defect suggests that the effective or successful use of these defense mechanisms, in warding off threat and anxiety, could *temporarily* serve a protective function, by maintaining emotional equilibrium. Repression and denial might well be maintained, even until the onset of symptoms of ARC or AIDS related illness, or evidence of T-cell loss from a blood-test.

The problem with the use of such defense mechanisms, however, is that, as they avoid confrontation with reality, failure or de-compensation of defenses may result in the loss of emotional equilibrium. Indeed, several studies have shown that it is such failure of a person's defense or coping mechanisms which results in pathophysiological changes, as pointed out, for example, by Solomon in the papers mentioned previously. In therapy, the learning of more reality-based, adaptive coping strategies, should probably be an important aim.

Finally, the link between suppression of depressed feelings and the presence of a defect in T-cell immunity, seems to be consistent with Bahnson's view, quoted above, concerning the repression of negative emotions and their discharging 'somatically, within the organism.' It is also consistent with the published data of Kissen, Greer, Magarey and Todd concerning associations between 'bottled-up' negative emotions, especially anger, and malignancy, specifically lung and breast cancer. However, the stage in disease process at which coping or defense mechanisms fail and negative emotional states surface, might well also be crucial to illness progression as well as to immune status. This issue, too, needs to be addressed in future research, particularly in longitudinal studies.

Conclusions

The results of this essentially exploratory study should be confirmed and extended in future longtitudinal investigations. However, the data already helps to suggest which personality, stress and emotional factors should be the targets of psychotherapeutic or counseling approaches with HIV infected persons. The importance of the data is perhaps underscored by its convergence and consistency with the results of studies of other immune-related diseases, suggesting the salience of the 'immunosuppression-prone personality pattern'.

Psychosocial interventions should aim to influence immunity and the course of disease, as well as quality of life and well-being, and must, of course, be evaluated in controlled studies. The next chapter discusses how such approaches as psychotherapy, counseling and creative visualization might be used to try to influence immunity and illness in HIV infection. A primary aim would be to prevent the onset of AIDS spectrum disorders with early interventions. The later in the course of HIV infection such interventions are implemented, the less is the likelihood of making a significant difference to the disease process, a proposition supported by Levy's work on psychosocial factors in late or advanced stages of cancer.

Finally, scientific data such as that reported here, represents a challenge to moral theology. Only insofar as scientific understanding of such matters as the homosexual condition is integrated into theology, can genuine reconciliation and healing be accomplished.

CHAPTER FIVE

Therapies: How Might We Modify Immunity and Illness?

Statistics from the 1987 Washington AIDS Conference suggested that about 36 per cent of HIV infected persons will eventually develop full-blown or terminal AIDS. Later studies have been much less sanguine, with estimates of up to 90 per cent or beyond progressing to terminal illness. It is currently believed that some 60,000 to 90,000 individuals in Australia are already HIV antibody positive. More than 16,000 cases have actually tested as HIV infected.

However, the grimmer estimates of proportions of infected persons progressing to AIDS assume *an absence of interventions* which might significantly influence immunity and the course of disease. Current data in psychoneuroimmunology suggests that much could be done, using psychological techniques, to reduce the incidence of AIDS, even among persons already infected or with early symptoms, for example of ARC. Such a potential for influencing or decelerating the course of infection is over and beyond the value of such strategies in enhancing quality of life and well-being, important as these aims are.

If this claim is valid, then the relief of human suffering, morbidity and mortality, as well as the reduction in the drain on the public purse could be monumental indeed!

What Needs to Change?

As we have seen, current research data supports the validity of the concept of an 'immunosuppression-prone personality pattern,' relevant to autoimmune disorders and infections, including now HIV. The factors which should be the targets of psychosocial interventions, on the basis of this evidence, are: (a) 'bottled-up' or suppressed negative emotions, especially anger and rage; (b) conflicts about homosexual identity; (c) coping with loss; (d) defense or coping mechanisms promoting emotional equilibrium; (e) depression; (f) perceived control (personal power) over health status; (g) internalized stigma (homophobia); (h) inward-turning anger (self-hatred); (i) social support and (j) the spiritual dimension of meaning and commitment.

Psychotherapy, counseling and other techniques should ideally focus upon modifying these sorts of factors, as early as possible after infection with HIV. This is the goal of *secondary prevention* and one which so far has been minimized in importance in treatment. It is likely that ignorance of psychoneuroimmunological data and entrenched medical-model attitudes and conservatism have contributed to this neglect.

Group Learning

Even while agreeing about the factors to be changed on the basis of existing scientific evidence, therapists and counselors will naturally differ somewhat in the methods they use to influence these factors. However, most would probably concur that both psychodynamic and cognitive-behavioural techniques are important. This is the spirit of eclecticism! Creative visualization and meditation methods, described later as adjuncts to psychotherapy, also appear to be valuable and are summed up in the papers of Delmonte, Kutz and Magarey listed in the Bibliography.

In my opinion, the best work can be done in groups of eight to twelve persons, carefully assessed and meeting at least weekly, for twelve or more weeks. Preliminary observations suggest that changes in both psychological factors and immune factors can occur within such timeframes, although this impression needs to be confirmed. Such group participation immediately reduces social isolation and allows for the testing out of self-concepts as well as the open expression and sharing of fears, concerns and feelings. Group members are asked to agree to complete confidentiality of what is disclosed in the group, creating a climate of safety, trust and emotional support. This facilitates the letting go of defensiveness and the building of emotional bonds.

Preventing Suicide

One aspect of group work which may be overlooked is the value of emotional support and of the constructive working through of negative emotions such as rage and depression and conflicts about loss and sexual identity in preventing self-destructive behaviour and suicide.

Early after diagnosis of HIV antibody positive status or ARC symptoms, many people regress emotionally. This means they become vulnerable, dependent and frightened as they confront the implications of diagnosis. Depression, understood as inward-turning anger or rage and as a stage of grieving, is very common and suicidal ideas or frank attempts are frequent. What is to be done?

We should remind ourselves that patients become angry not only about loss, mortality and other implications of diagnosis, but also, in view of the emotional regression, about *past* experiences of loss and issues about homosexual identity or 'coming-out' which are re-awakened at this time. They are frequently angry with their partners and other significant persons. Suicidal behaviour, in this context, may be understood as an unconscious homicide, the symbolic killing of an internalized other person.

Support, and especially the ventilation of intense, 'irrational' emotions such as rage, are likely to reduce the risk of suicide and other self-destructive behaviours such as alcohol or drug abuse. It is well-known that such substance abuse is commonly a passive or indirect expression of suicidal impulses. It is also likely to be immunosuppressive.

What Happens in a Group?

Typically, in the first couple of sessions, members share experiences concerns and issues related to positive HIV antibody status. This results in much mutual 'mirroring' and in the discovery of common themes. Barriers and the common feeling of being 'untouchable' or stigmatized, as well as the tendency to isolate, are replaced with a growing openness, reduced loneliness and an enhanced courage in exploring painful conflicts and (sometimes terrifying) emotions.

Later, the mirroring process deepens and helps in the reliving of buried or unconscious memories, emotions and conflicts, re-awakened in the present, often due to the impact of HIV antibody positive diagnosis. This usually results in a re-surfacing of issues about sexual identity, coming-out, stigma, loss, mortality, difficulties in forming lasting emotional bonds, trust and morbid jealousy.

Analysis (interpretation) of such 'transference-like' responses, that is, misperceiving the present in terms of the past, is a vital part of group psychotherapy which goes far beyond what is attempted in simple support groups. This work is consistent with the emphasis of Bahnson and others upon the importance of resolving, 'core psychodynamic conflicts' and is probably necessary for healing and personal growth, as well as the enrichment of subsequent relationships.

However, such deep interventions should be used only

by trained health professionals who have had some supervized experience in psychotherapy, as well as coursework in relevant theory. Persons without such training are likely to personalize transference reactions directed towards them, reacting instead of understanding what is happening as a part of a group process necessary to effective therapy and lasting change. In other words, the counselor's own unresolved issues tend to get in the way, as these are mirrored by patients and especially if the therapist or counselor is HIV antibody positive. I explore this question more thoroughly in chapter seven, under the heading of 'counter transference'.

Group members also learn to become less guarded and more emotionally expressive instead of bottling-up feelings such as anger. Instead, they are given training in assertiveness and in positive emotional expressiveness. This helps to overcome the tabooing of tenderness and affection, often a big problem for males in our culture.

Inward-turning anger (self-hatred) is reversed in the process of reappraising self-images (often projected onto others and therefore not acknowledged). This reversal may aid in the enrichment of relationships, as individuals become more self-accepting and forgiving of themselves and others.

Powerlessness is gradually replaced with a sense of control over and responsibility for one's own health and that of others. This change occurs through commitment to the group work (doing something constructive) as well as through active involvement in other growth-promoting and health-enhancing activities.

Creative Visualization

The use of creative visualization and meditation as adjuncts to group psychotherapy or counselling has been described by several writers, including Delmonte, Kutz and Magarey. Visualizations are best given after deep relaxation or hypnotic induction and consist largely of images and metaphors about the immune system and healing. They often help patients get in touch with feelings and issues surfacing in group psychotherapeutic sessions.

Associate Professor Wendy Walker believes that the effectiveness of trance, as well as visualization and suggestion, is enhanced through the use of suitable music. She also suspects that the use of such methods may be immuno-facilitating, that is, tending to boost immunity, such as increasing the production of T-cells or natural killer cell activity, although this attractive notion needs to be evaluated through controlled research. There is little doubt, however, that subjective well-being and the experience of positive emotional states such as joy and delight as well as quality of life can be enhanced markedly!

More will be said about the value of these techniques, later, as possible means of awakening meaning and spirituality, and some examples are given in Part Four of this book.

CHAPTER SIX

A Long Night's Journey into Day

ISSUES FOR THERAPISTS COUNSELORS, CLERGY AND CARERS

The Therapist's Perspective

Therapeutic work with people facing life-threatening illnesses or at risk of developing such conditions requires a unique perspective. *Timeframes* are critical, as the group work must effect changes and facilitate the crossing of thresholds of healing and recovery as quickly as possible. In the pilgrimage towards healing, both the guides (therapists) and the pilgrims (patients) set out to combat the biological consequences of exposure to a virus which leaves infected persons with gravely breached defences against various opportunistic infections and malignancy. Time is of the essence!

It is essential also that interventions are *focused*. This means working on the psychological factors known to influence both immunity and the disease process. Thus, psychotherapy and counseling for HIV infected persons is different in duration and content from traditional approaches relevant to neuroses or to problems in living.

Experience of working with HIV infected persons reveals several issues which must be addressed by health professionals and community carers if they are to remain both effective in their roles and well themselves. The first of these issues arises from the uncanny 'mirroring' of emotional material which occurs as we accompany patients on the pathway to recovery.

Countertransference

The mirroring of our own unconscious issues, conflicts and emotions in work with patients is referred to technically as *countertransference*. To achieve insight into this reality and to enhance our own coping and effectiveness, we need to take 'a long night's journey into day,' a journey into the unconscious, to discover our own defenses, blind-spots and hidden conflicts, especially concerning mortality and sexual identity.

In working with HIV infected persons, the experience of countertransference can be extremely powerful. This reflects the fact that patients resemble us in so many ways, sharing similar lifestyles and values, sometimes being about the same age and socioeconomic status. Thus patients can very easily mirror unresolved issues we may face about loss, mortality and sexual identity. Moreover, loss of such patients through death can be particularly devastating, as *over-identification* may intensify and complicate the grieving process. Each loss can represent our own death! Under these circumstances, multiple losses and so-called 'bereavement-overload' can contribute to rapid burn out.

How then do we learn to recognize countertransference and to correct for it, so that it does not get in the way of effective therapeutic work? Symptoms include inappropriate emotional reactions which are disproportionate in intensity or are clearly a reflection of some issue within ourselves. We may find ourselves devoting excessive time to some patient at the expense of others and rationalizing such responses, although their inappropriateness will be obvious to other sensitive, trained people.

Another sign is a growing feeling of indispensability and the fantasy that no-one else could possibly be of as much assistance to 'our' patients. Some patients, too, become symbolically significant to us, and working though our dreams and fantasies can be of help in recognizing when particular persons have acquired such meaning for us.

The existence of countertransference is, in a sense, a caricature of something valuable. That is our capacity for 'projective identification' or empathy. However, if left unmonitored, it can reduce our competence and effectiveness markedly. The complications arising from countertransference are a further cogent reason for specialized training and supervision of health professionals and carers, especially early in their work with HIV infected persons.

Experienced therapists and counselors should review their own emotional responses regularly with colleagues; especially after loss. A lack of suitable training, supervision and support is a recipe for *burn out*.

Preventing Burn Out

The symptoms of burn out include emotional blunting (numbness, apathy), depression, irritability, insomnia, substance abuse (alcohol, sedatives), reduced empathy, feelings of indispensability and denial of diminishing competence. Its toll can be devastating for both health professionals and for patients. However, prevention is possible.

Possible preventive measures include: (a) 'time-out' and extra stress leave; (b) trained and supervised experience; (c) the personal experience of psychotherapy; (d) support, de-briefing and consultation to aid in the monitoring of countertransference issues; (e) reviewing case-loads; (f) grief counseling to counter bereavement overload; (g) periods of time spent on teaching or research or working with patients who are not seriously ill or terminal and (h) regular meditation practice and exercise.

Expecting health professionals and community carers to cope and to function effectively without adequate support, supervision and consultation from other skilled persons is unrealistic and destructive, compounding the stresses contributing to burn out, such as isolation and bottled-up emotions. The role of group dynamics and personality factors within the social systems providing health care for HIV infected persons must also be addressed and understood. Victim-blaming is not a solution to the problem of burn out. The emphasis must be upon compassion, and understanding of the causes, prevention and treatment.

Training

If the remarkable potential of psychological and spiritual approaches to healing is to be realized fully, adequate training of health professionals and community carers is vital. Such persons need to acquire knowledge of the implications of research in psychosomatic medicine and psychoneuroimmunology and expertise in relevant therapeutic skills. This is, of course, the inspiration for this book! Such persons also require ongoing supervision, support and the opportunity to resolve issues arising from counter-transference, grieving and other stressors.

Often, those involved in this work are unaware of relevant research data and many also lack appropriate training in psychotherapeutic or counseling skills relevant to work with HIV infected persons. Such gaps cannot be filled by viewing a few video tapes or attending a workshop or two, although such experiences are valuable. Further, the view that so-called 'peer-group support' is all that is required is an absurd pretence, given the growing scientific knowledge about psychological factors influencing immunity and illness and the need for considerable expertise in appropriate strategies for modifying such factors.

It is time for a radical reappraisal of objectives and priorities within the health care systems and community organizations concerned with AIDS. Perhaps too, the focus needs to be increasingly upon how to *enhance living with dignity and personal growth as well as the prevention of illness in HIV antibody positive persons, rather than upon death and dying only.* For the message of psychoneuroimmunological data is one of realistic optimism and hope!

CHAPTER SEVEN

Awakening Meaning: The Spiritual Dimension of Healing

Albert Camus, in *The Myth of Sisyphus*, reminds us of a cosmic image of futility. Sisyphus was the figure condemned for all eternity to roll a rock uphill, only to have it roll back down again. It would be difficult to imagine a more compelling archetype or universal symbol of frustration and meaninglessness. It is precisely the belief that our lives are ultimately futile that can raise doubts about going on—especially when facing the grim realities of HIV infection. It is perhaps a supreme irony that, as Viktor Frankl, the Viennese psychiatrist interned in Auschwitz, has pointed out in his book, *Man's Search for Meaning*, merely *prolonging* an apparently futile life, does not in itself confer meaning. Purpose and meaning flow from a changed perception of who we are and can become. Meaning thus begins with a spiritual awakening and with the emergence of values. It often implies a 'death' of one's ego, to allow for the experience of a deeper self or higher power or of what Frankl terms one's 'unconscious God'. This symbolic death of the ego is relative and implies acknowledgement of a transcendent reality, not annihilation of the ego itself.

Suicide: Option or Opting Out?

In the Nazi concentration camps, meaning could no longer arise either from an illusion of immortality (denial of death) or from the belief that life might be extended indefinitely. Death could and often did come at sudden, unexpected moments. Meaning could only be realized hour by hour.

For some inmates, it stemmed from an awareness of incompleted tasks (unfinished business). For others it was care for a loved one or even belief in a personal God to whom one felt responsible. Once, after witnessing the hanging of a prisoner, one inmate answered the despairing cry, 'Where is God now?' with the statement, 'He is there, suspended from the rope!'

Meaning lay in sunsets or in sharing one's last piece of bread with another prisoner—'communion' in the deepest human sense. Those who found no meaning usually died of an immune-related illness (infection) or committed suicide by running into an electrified wire.

In HIV infection, patients often experience a similar, sudden change in their perception of time and meaning. Faced with the real possibility of developing AIDS, the question arises: 'If I am to lose much or all of the things, in terms of which I have defined myself (sexuality, career, status, body-image, etc.) what meaning could the rest of my life have? Why go on? Why *be*?'

Awakening Meaning

In psychotherapeutic or counseling groups for HIV antibody positive persons, these issues must be addressed, usually in the context of working through questions about personal identity and self-worth. The question, 'Who am I?' becomes intimately linked with another: 'Why would I *not* commit suicide?'

Some individuals provide hints of their answers indirectly. For example, a recent history of drug or alcohol abuse suggests immediately a thinly-veiled self-destructiveness, or a tendency towards slow suicide. This occurs in a context of denial or ambivalence about going on. The balance between the will to live and the unconscious wish to die is fine and the scales need to be tipped urgently!

Those who cannot answer the question at all or who stammer out phony, hollow replies are usually very vulnerable. They may be at risk for more serious suicide attempts. The issue in therapy becomes that of how to *awaken meaning*—how to tip the balance. One key lies in changing the person's focus from a concern with mere quantity of life to an emphasis upon quality and the realization of values as well as neglected growth potential in the here and now. In this context, illness can be redefined as an opportunity for transformation and a change of direction in life.

It is also vital to help patients to achieve insight into unconscious fantasies which may be translated into self-destructive behaviour. For example, many patients unconsciously wish to be re-united with recently lost partners or, through buried guilt, wish to punish themselves. Understanding the role of anger is important here. Suicide is frequently an unconscious *homicide*, the symbolic killing of an internalized other. Karl Menninger in his book *Man Against Himself* coined the term 'somatic suicide' to refer to the role of repressed rage in the development of life-threatening illnesses such as cancer. The term is equally apt when applied to other passive suicidal methods.

The Value of Groups

Psychotherapeutic or counseling groups for HIV infected persons can save valuable lives as well as being means of preventing illness and of awakening meaning. Suicidism is quite common early after diagnosis.

Firstly, such groups offer emotional support during the painful process of confronting issues such as real or threatened loss, identity, sexuality, rage, powerlessness and spirituality. Secondly, members learn to work through scary, sometimes terrifying emotions, conflicts and loneliness in a setting of mutual care, respect, nurture and acceptance. The early exchange of telephone numbers, and simply *being there* for one another, facilitate this process, while also encouraging a move away from tortured self-concern and the common tendency to isolate oneself. These elements, too, are essential for healing, growth and the experience of meaning and commitment to others.

Meditation and Creative Visualization

The use of meditation and visualization as adjuncts to psychotherapy seems to have enormous potential. Both techniques help people to get in touch with buried emotions and deeper aspects of identity as well as awakening the spiritual dimension of recovery and healing. Many writers have described these techniques in detail, including Delmonte, Kutz and Magarey and I provide some examples in chapters eleven and twelve.

Some visualizations are metaphors and images about the immune system and healing. Others aim to induce the letting go of negative emotions and to enhance the experience of relatively pure active-positive emotions such as joy and delight and other feelings flowing from what are called 'peak identity experiences'. In these experiences, the conscious ego is overcome by or suspended in a remarkably pure perception of deeper aspects of the self, of the ground of one's being or of one's 'unconscious God'. Linked with them also is an awareness of apparently universal truths, of what Carl Jung calls archetypal symbols (see, for example, *Psychology and Religion: West and East*).

The accompanying emotions are a combination of awe, humility, serenity and, sometimes, ecstasy. Loss of the fear of death is particularly common, together with the discovery of previously unsuspected or neglected possibilities for personal growth and creativity. Clinical work with cancer patients suggests that such experiences might well enhance survival time, though such claims must be evaluated in controlled studies.

I suspect that these 'mystical' or peak experiences might represent thresholds of healing and recovery, although this hunch, too, needs to be tested. At the very least, the use of visualization and meditation should result in greatly enhanced well-being and vitality as well as improved quality of life in HIV infected persons.

A Higher Power or Deeper Self

The concept of a spiritual reality, personal God or higher Power is a difficult one for many patients because of unfortunate experiences with orthodox religions. Some persons who have abandoned institutionalized religious structures have not discovered any deeper spiritual dimension and may be bankrupt of meaning or commitment to any sort of larger social-cultural-spiritual whole. Western society tends to be obsessed with materialism and with self-definition in terms of amassing possessions and power. Thus the real or threatened loss of these things can be profoundly devastating. However, such loss may also be an opportunity for deeper self discovery and personal transformation.

The result of our obsession with materialism and power can be alienation from ourselves and from others, as Erich Fromm has pointed out in his book *The Sane Society*. In Western society, a cult of egoism and self-centredness has created cynicism and spiritual bankruptcy on a mass collective scale.

However, the process of personal growth and healing seems to entail a move away from this self-centred predicament. This is coupled with a move towards self-transcendence, that is, being in contact with some form of deeper spiritual reality or higher power. This might be a subculture, community, the human-species or a personal God. Commitment and responsibility to a larger whole, beyond one's ego, is the essential element.

Much religious symbolism and ritual are collective means of facilitating the development of conscious contact with this transcendent function or reality. According to Jung, historically the great religious systems have been both the matrix or source and the means of awakening what he describes as the archetypal or universal symbols of full selfhood, humanness and healing.

In summary, at some point of the pilgrimage to healing and growth or transformation, one discovers something or *someone* to whom one feels responsible, and this reality is not the ego. It is in fact, the deepest self and the person's unrealized possibilities for creativity and growth—for fullest humanness. The humanistic psychologists such as Maslow refer to this process as 'self-actualization'.

The discovery is one of the most moving experiences of identity-formation and is associated with awe, humility and, sometimes, sheer fright! For St Francis of Assisi, it was a voice in a ruined church, (unconscious) symbol of his spiritual bankruptcy, saying, 'Go, repair My house,' and meaning, 'Your body is My temple, so stop destroying it!'

For those who have reported near-death experiences, this experience is often expressed as a sense of tasks incompleted and of authentic guilt about wasting time and talents which could be used for the good of others. After such remarkable experiences, life for these persons assumes an added dimension of richness and meaning. The focus is upon realizing the creative possibilities of each moment—*as if it could be one's last*.

Ultimately, suicide is *not* the answer to the question 'Why be?' It is in fact a flight into absurdity, analogous to solving a problem in chess by simply sweeping the pieces off the board. It is the final, irrevocable cop-out. Only when one's condition is *truly terminal* does the option of not taking medications or of not accepting heroic life-support measures become a valid one. Perhaps then, but only then, might such a gesture be a final gift of love.

Pastoral Care

The techniques outlined briefly in this chapter are probably equally relevant to professional therapists, counselors, clergy and community carers. However, clergy, priests, ministers and rabbis—professional religious persons—also have access to sacramental and to other powerful symbolic means of facilitating inner wholeness and healing. The origins of such means of grace and spiritual healing lie deep in history and their efficacy comes from truly archetypal processes at work in the human psyche—as suggested decades ago by Carl Jung.

The healing of memories and the use of the sacramental means of promoting inner reconciliation and wholeness, as well as counseling, do fall into the domain of pastoral care. As living 'icons of Christ', priests can do much to cleanse away and to relieve people living with HIV/AIDS of much morbid stigma, guilt, self-hatred and depression and therefore, of considerable inner 'dis-ease' with self. However, to fulfil such a role, priests themselves need to have encountered the Shadow and to have dealt with issues of human mortality and sexuality. They must be willing to experience the inner journey towards wholeness and this can mean the experience of something like crucifixion, a ritual dis-memberment, on a symbolic and emotional level.

PART THREE

AIDS AND COMMUNITY GROWTH

CHAPTER EIGHT

The Issue of Screening and the Educational Challenge

To Be Tested or not to Be Tested?

Screening for exposure to the human immunodeficiency virus (HIV) in at-risk groups is usually justified on the grounds that knowledge of antibody status should result in precautions to avoid infection of others. Thus, the adoption of so-called 'safe sexual practices', including condom usage, is recommended, perhaps with some suggestions about lifestyle changes, such as cutting back on alcohol and drugs and reducing stress levels.

However, such advice rests upon the naive assumption that people will necessarily respond rationally to factual information, by modifying high-risk behaviours—a dubious assumption, for reasons discussed below. Perhaps the most powerful argument for antibody testing is largely overlooked. This is the claim that knowing one's antibody status can help a person to regain a sense of control and to reduce helplessness by doing something active to minimize the likelihood of becoming ill once exposed to HIV. The research described in this book on linkages between psychological factors, immunity and disease, as well as concepts of effective intervention, support this goal of *secondary prevention* of illness—over and beyond the availability of chemotherapy, in the form of drugs such as AZT and

DDI, and the use of antibiotics to minimize the risk of pneumocystis pneumonia.

Participation in groups providing psychotherapy, counseling, meditation and creative visualization facilitates the development of a sense of being in control over or responsible for one's health as well as enhancing well-being and quality of life. If psychological factors do in fact account for about half of the individual variation in whether or not people develop T-cell immune defects as well as predicting illness onset, such group work might well also influence the course of infection itself.

Thus the message to communicate in media campaigns and educational programs aiming to change high-risk behaviours is that individuals can regain control and care for themselves and others by presenting for screening and through active involvement in appropriate therapeutic or counseling programs, as well as medical treatment.

The decision *not* to be tested reflects fear, defensiveness (denial) and perceived lack of control over AIDS, among other motivational factors. Fear-arousing messages, such as those communicated in the Grim Reaper commercials, seem likely to compound resistances to screening, at least among persons whose characteristic defences against threat are avoidance mechanisms such as denial or repression. The research data on behaviours related to other life-threatening illnesses such as cancer support this claim and are summarized in many papers, including my article entitled, 'Ego-Defences and Affects in Women with Breast Symptoms: A Preliminary Measurement Paradigm' (see Bibliography). The influence of unconscious motives represents a true challenge for health educators and health care planners.

The Educational Challenge

Teachers have a unique opportunity to model positive attitudes as well as the task of disseminating accurate factual information about AIDS and human sexuality. For it is within our education system that myths and misinformation can be most easily corrected in the light of solid, scientific evidence.

Judd Marmor, in *Homosexual Behaviour: A Modern Reappraisal*, has compiled a set of papers which sum up what is currently known about the development of sexual identity and gender roles as well as negative, self-hating attitudes and destructive behaviour patterns. Social change, in the sense of cultivating attitudes of tolerance, understanding and compassion, must begin with our children. This educational challenge has been recognized by many individuals, but still seems to be avoided by some administrators with conservative or homophobic attitudes.

The situation with respect to AIDS and human sexuality is simply a special case of the more general social problem of teaching understanding of the origins of prejudice and the dynamics of minority group oppression. The solution will be as relevant to promoting the growth and well-being of racial minorities, for example, as to that of persons at risk of HIV infections or AIDS. *Homophobia is of the same nature and has its roots in the same psychic factors as does racial prejudice and its effects are equally damaging.*

Prejudice and oppression not only perpetuate social injustice, but they also result in much psychological morbidity, reflecting the internalization of stigma and the development of self-hating attitudes in affected persons. The unconscious choice of negative identity and the acting-out of rage in antisocial behaviour are other effects. We now know also that such attitudes increase the proneness to illness, including AIDS.

The educational challenge represents another dimension of the social transformation that is required if we are to create a truly pluralistic, multicultural society with genuine freedom and respect for the rights of all persons. AIDS confronts us collectively with the necessity of addressing and responding to this challenge.

The Role of the Churches

It could be suggested of those Christians with more extreme fundamentalist attitudes towards HIV/AIDS and homosexuality that if a serpent looks into the mirror of the scriptures, it cannot expect to see the image of an angel reflected back. Such people not only tend to ignore science, they also neglect to consider the historical, cultural and sociological contexts in which the scriptures were written—interpreting the biblical references to such issues as homosexuality from a position of literalism and gross ignorance.

Fundamentalists also tend to be afraid of their 'shadows' (in Carl Jung's sense), and to be preoccupied with the specks in their brothers' or sisters' eyes while overlooking the beams in their own. Their contributions to the educational challenge of HIV/AIDS, especially in the mass-media, often reflect these limitations in perception and understanding.

The clergy, whether Catholic or Protestant, are human, and as a group are not immune to ignorance, fear and prejudice, especially about sexual matters. Their consciousness, of course, is shaped by the thought-patterns of particular historical and cultural situations; as was the mind of St Paul himself, who probably had no idea of the distinction between a homosexual condition or identity, which is discovered, and things 'perversely' chosen through acts of free will. Many, unfortunately, cling to medieval concepts of human sexuality, especially those expressed by St Thomas Aquinas in the *Summa Theologica*, written two centuries before the rise of empirical science. Again, their contributions, educationally and pastorally, tend to mirror these limitations in understanding.

The churches, with some exceptions, have integrated the results of scientific revolutions—other than that in the understanding of human sexuality—into their thinking. Many theologians happily quote nowadays from the works of Charles Darwin, Sigmund Freud, Carl Jung and other pioneers in the history of ideas. Neither the revolution of the earth around the sun, nor the evolution of species, as a mechanism of creation, have to be denied. It is perhaps time, in this era of AIDS, for modern scientific knowledge about such factual matters as homosexual identity formation to be taken seriously; even in theological training, at colleges and in seminaries. And science does reveal that homosexuality is intrinsic to the very being of millions of people —between five and ten percent of the population, according to the famous Kinsey Report estimates.

If the educational vision of the gospels, the 'good news' of the Christian message, is truly about becoming fully human and whole and about liberation from the bondage of oppression, then the churches might well adopt the posture of their founder towards those who continue to perpetuate the stigmatization and who therefore contribute to the suffering and ultimately to the killing of people living with HIV/AIDS, irrespective of their sexual orientation. Jesus healed the lepers, without asking that first they should repent, and to those who were worried about the 'sins' of the blind man his reply was 'What is that to you?' Who is without sin or a human shadow?

Finally, if one dimension of education is the influence of role models, then one might ask the more conservative members of the clergy whether, in view of the analyses of Freud and others of such historical figures as Michaelangelo and Leonardo da Vinci, children should be exposed to the artistic masterpieces created by these latent or overtly homosexual men? Perhaps, certain people would suggest whitewashing the Sistine Chapel or locking away the famous pieta and statue of David, lest these images corrupt the minds of our youth! Stated like this, the absurdity of such preoccupations is obvious indeed!

CHAPTER NINE

Transformation: Personal and Collective

The emergence of AIDS probably represents a turning point in human evolution. It is the first time in human history that a micro-organism has acquired the capacity to destroy its biological defence system. Overcoming AIDS will entail a *radical transformation* of attitudes and values at both personal and collective levels. Medical breakthroughs are unlikely to be sufficient and might well be many years in the future. These claims might be illuminated by briefly reflecting upon the role of humanity in cultural evolution.

A Vision of Past and Future

In and through human beings, evolution has become auto-evolution. No longer just the gradual effect of the natural selection of chance variations, the blind result of random mutations, evolution has become not only conscious of itself, but *directed*. This vision, shared by such eminent biologists as Julian Huxley and the Jesuit palaeontologist Teilhard de Chardin, confers upon us an awesome dignity and a unique responsibility. It is mirrored at both individual and collective levels and illuminates our future possibilities for growth, wholeness and tranformation, including the challenge of coping with and overcoming AIDS.

Wholeness

We confront a destiny made up of biological, psychological and social forces, to be shaped uniquely by each one of us. Thus we weave ourselves into the fabric of human history. We can achieve mastery and control over our lives, rather than experience events, including our health status, as merely due to chance, fate or the influence of powerful others.

Far from being merely statistical atoms, we are in fact centres of consciousness and reflection, drawn together by the irresistible attraction of loving energy. This binds us not only to those closest to us, but also to communities, subcultures, the whole human species. Personal growth reflects identification with and commitment to such larger wholes. Translating this identification into positive action is perhaps the ultimate expression of positive identity and wholeness.

Altered States

At a collective level, the slow dawning of a sense of species represents the rise of a striving, however subliminal at first, for the unanimization (literally, union of souls) of humankind, through universal aspirations and shared love. Utopian? Perhaps, but a hint of this future 'altered state' already exists, I believe, in certain communities of scientists and in some spiritual movements.

A longing for its realization was probably present in such visionaries as Ghandi, Einstein and Pope John XXIII. The latter individual deplored the splits in Christianity and began a slow process of reconciliation and healing through the Second Vatican Council.

The spiritual awakening I am referring to is not simply a push for collectivization as conceived by Marxists. It is rather the unfolding of a global consciousness and a universal embrace of all in and through a personal centre. As Teilhard de Chardin put it, *Erit in omnibus, omnia Deus*, which means, 'God in all through all'. In short, what the visionaries seem to be getting at is the possibility of a truly 'mystical' union, in which both personal growth and a contribution to a larger social-cultural-spiritual whole are perfectly compatible.

Such a view is also quite consistent with the holistic model of healing and illness described in this book. Holism implies perceiving illnesses and the process of healing as involving the total system of human beings and their environment—the full *biopsychosocial* reality of the human condition.

Personal Transformation

To put some flesh on the bones of what may seem like a very speculative view, I would like in this chapter to describe a little of my own personal experience of spiritual transformation, as a prelude to discussing such changes at a collective level and in more general terms. My intention is to share something of the hope and confidence which I now believe such a world-view inspires. It is simply a confession of faith!

My early background was in the type of Irish orthodox Catholic tradition described by James Joyce in *Portrait of the Artist as a Young Man*, or portrayed with refreshing humour in Fred Schepisi's film *The Devil's Playground*. This form of Roman Catholicism was strongly influenced by Jansenist ideas of 'sin' and 'unworthiness'. It promoted in me a morbid scrupulosity, as well as a rather joyless, intense attitude to life—religiosity or pietism, not genuine spirituality. Little wonder if life was a minefield of possibilities for mortal sin and the horrors of eternal damnation!

My awakening sexuality was riddled with fear and guilt. It was therefore denied and disowned for most of my adolescence and early adulthood. During my undergraduate years at Sydney University, the entire edifice of Catholic belief began to collapse. Exposed to the philosophy of the logical positivitists and the rigors of behaviourism in Psychology, I finally became a convinced atheist.

Soon I also became hedonistic, grossly self-centred and spiritually bankrupt. When it surfaced, my sexuality was compulsive, isolated from the rest of my personality and exploitative. Personal transformation was needed for full integration of my sexuality and for the development of a genuine capacity for loving myself and others. How could the sexuality which I had painfully discovered within myself, not freely chosen, be put together with feeling and spirituality?

Encounter with Death

The first step in my spiritual awakening was quite sudden. In some ways it was like Paul's conversion on the road to Damascus. I was literally struck down with a serious heart condition. Faced with possible death, I became painfully aware of deserts of wasted opportunity. Every moment became precious and daily events like sunsets took on a new freshness, as though experienced with the rapture and innocence of childhood. My own illusion that life might extend indefinitely into the future was shattered and my perception of time changed, so that I became very much oriented to the here and now.

More importantly, I became aware of tasks to fulfil, of *being questioned by the future*. A deep need arose to use my talents to do something about social change, oppression, bigotry and prejudice. My professional work took on a new meaning and became a source of 'peak experiences', no longer activities pursued for purely egoistic ends. Scientific discovery through research became a source of awe and humility before the complex mystery of the human person. Clinical encounters with others reflected a growing awareness of the extraordinary beauty, dignity and growth-

The Transcendent

So far, I had been given a new grasp of the meaning of 'scientific humanism'. However, subliminally, something still seemed to be missing. This was the deeper spiritual dimension of the mystical, the transcendent. Burn out was to set the stage for a more profound conversion. I was still full of intellectual reservations and, like St Augustine, unwilling and too proud to surrender totally. I trembled before the absurd.

Burn out, precipitated by multiple losses and other stresses, had led to my becoming addicted to sedatives. I was rapidly ceasing to be either effective or fully alive. Survival demanded that I get in touch with deeper aspects of my self, my 'unconscious God', in Frankl's terms. Recovery, quite early, resulted in moving insights into the personal significance of Jung's concepts of Christ as a symbol of the deeper self, of wholeness and integration of one's personality.

In the dark night of burn out, my ego and hubris died and true selfhood began to be born. The liturgy of the Catholic church, coupled with meditation, became a pathway to the experience of serenity, joy and self-transcendence. I had surrendered and discovered something of the capacity for empathy, creativity, humor and wisdom which such Jungians as Jacoby associate with individuation and wholeness.

The Veils Lift

If, as Teilhard de Chardin supposed, evolution is the unfolding of a 'noosphere', a global membrane of meaning, then the process must also have *direction*. It must also be a movement towards something or perhaps *someone*. Teilhard described this as 'Christogenesis'. However, he was simply expressing in theological terms his belief that God, as a spiritual reality, is both immanent (within all) and transcendent (beyond and embracing all).

These days my work, I hope, reflects a recognition of the spiritual dimension of humanity. If, as Carl Jung believed, the causes of possible global annihilation as well as factors contributing to disease, lie within the human psyche, then we must take psychological and spiritual issues seriously.

However, ==spirituality will be expressed in very diverse ways, depending upon a person's culture and early background.== Such individual differences must be respected and spiritual growth will be facilitated by a range of approaches, not just those associated with Western religious systems. Yet behind the rich diversity, as Jung has pointed out, lies a common, primal core of spiritual striving, expressed in universal, archetypal symbols of re-birth and wholeness, present, it seems, in all known human cultures.

Narcosis or Mystery?

Karl Marx once described religion as 'the opium of the people'. He was referring to the seductive certainties and numbing of free thought which he believed were characteristics of followers. His views might well be true for rigid and insecure persons and his insight into the abuse of religious ideologies for the propping up of oppressive political systems were, I believe, accurate.

However, for the open-minded and curious, spiritual values provide frameworks within which to contemplate and to grasp the many unsolved puzzles, the mystery, of the ascent of humanity in evolution. Such values also cast light upon the perplexing problems of evil and suffering.

Suffering and pain, for example, can be perceived as

disasters, devoid of meaning, or alternatively as opportunities for growth and change. Viktor Frankl has described this view eloquently in the context of commenting upon the qualities of survivors in the Nazi concentration camps. Psychosocial cancer research has also revealed much about the characteristics of long survivors and one objective of psychotherapy might well be that of helping HIV infected persons to acquire these vital qualities.

Perhaps, too, this is another perspective within which to perceive AIDS. Might it not be both a challenge to survival and a signpost to personal and collective growth and transformation? Certainly, clinical observation suggests that healing and recovery are reflected in a perception of regained control or personal power as well as an awakened sense of positive identity, meaning and commitment.

Growth observed in individual persons could be mirrored in collective, social changes, in the transformation of social systems and community organizations concerned with AIDS. The next chapter explores some of the changes which appear to be taking place in attitudes towards sexuality and relationships. This area, of course, is ripe for study by social scientists and theologians.

CHAPTER TEN

Relationships: Integrating Sexuality and Spirituality

In response to the AIDS crisis, a collective reappraisal of the quality and meaning of relationships is long overdue. Indeed, observation of the beginnings of such a process in society suggests that as part of this re-evaluation we might be witnessing a renaissance of commitment. If so, such a shift in consciousness could be significant to all persons irrespective of their sexual preferences. Many heterosexual as well as homosexual people seem to be adrift in a sea of uncertainty about such issues as monogamy and commitment. This chapter explores attitudes towards sexuality and relationships and the possibilities for reappraisal and growth as well as enrichment.

Safe Sex and Commitment

The adoption of 'safe sexual practices' is presently advocated in the light of epidemiological research data on the pathways by which the human immunodeficiency virus (HIV) is transmitted. However, such recommendations frequently ignore the fact that simply informing people about high-risk behaviour may not be sufficient to induce change. This is the conclusion to be drawn from decades of research on attitudes and behaviour related to life-threatening illnesses generally. Such advice does not usually address the complex issue of *motivation*, referred to in chapter nine (see pages 68–9).

Sexual behaviour, risky or otherwise, reflects many powerful emotional factors. These include the use of defences such as denial, the acting-out of repressed anger and depression, perceived personal power or control over life events and, of course, the need for intimacy and affection.

Most of these factors are non-rational and beyond conscious awareness and control. Risky or unsafe sexual practices and promiscuity often also represent responses to perceived oppression, self-hatred and unresolved issues concerning intimacy, bonding and trust. Such behaviours, therefore, are *not* easily susceptible to change simply by disseminating factual information.

Sometimes, the focus upon safe sex tends to divorce sexuality from the rest of the personality, perpetuating a process observed in both heterosexual and homosexual men of splitting off sexuality from the self concept as well as from emotions and spirituality. The question of forming relationships between *whole* persons, based upon mutual care, responsibility, respect and commitment is left totally unanswered.

People as Objects

Early socialization experiences in our culture lead many homosexuals to deny, disown or to split off their sexuality from the rest of their personalities. As pointed out by Vivienne Cass and others in papers on homosexual identity-formation, sexuality may be experienced by these people as something alien. Especially during the painful 'coming-out' process, partners tend to be perceived as objects, like vending machines, of little value in themselves and quite interchangable, provided they possess qualities or 'products' attractive on the personality or body markets.

This only intensifies self-alienation and the underlying sense that one is worthless or defaced—as proposed of homosexual people by many fundamentalists. Homophobia is internalized and perpetuated in acts of rebellion and illusory freedom. Many homosexual men in this situation don't bother talking to those who do not 'turn them on' and sexual encounters tend to be anonymous. Sometimes, these experiences are also repressed or forgotten, especially if the person is intoxicated.

The motivation is that of trying to pass as 'straight', in a context of partial denial of homosexual identity. The camouflage or self-deception can be both subtle and elaborate, but while protecting the person from painful feelings of shame and anxiety, it serves ultimately to delay acceptance of a positive sense of sexual identity. Fixation at early stages of homosexual identity-formation also precludes the possibility of loving and the full expression of needs for emotional intimacy. I have discussed the significance of non-acceptance of homosexual identity and diminished outlets for emotional expression for immunity and illness in HIV infection, earlier in chapter four (pages 35–7). Such unresolved issues probably enhance biological vulnerability to HIV!

Bonding and Intimacy

During childhood, many later homosexual persons have felt 'different' and become locked into emotional isolation. This has resulted from difficulties in bonding, poor role-modelling, pathological family psychodynamics and a conspicuous absence of positive homosexual or bisexual role models. Clinically, such individuals often present with severe disturbances in object relationships as defined by Winnicott (1989).

Coupled with learning experiences which conveyed the message that a homosexual preference was itself a symptom of maladjustment or immoral, such bonding difficulties frequently resulted in denial or disowning of a vital dimension of personality, with disastrous consequences for later adult relationships as well as mental and physical health and well-being.

For such people, then, adult relationships tend to be characterized by excessive mistrust, anxiety and projected self-hatred. The tendency to perceive people as objects has already been discussed. In the end, many homosexual men cannot love others because they are not yet capable of accepting and loving themselves and the underlying causes are largely unconscious. This plight also leaves them very vulnerable to illness, and is probably reflected in a high incidence of alcoholism and drug addiction in the homosexual community.

Morbid Jealousy

Silverstein, in his book, *Man to Man*, has pointed out that difficulties with bonding, insecurity, fear and possessiveness, in conjunction with projection onto others of homophobic, self-hating attitudes, can reach the level of paranoia and morbid jealousy. Such jealousy usually reflects irrational, unconscious fears about infidelity which are rooted in underlying issues about loss, separation and abandonment, as well as a sense of worthlessness and guilt.

One or both partners may feel emotionally suffocated. Instead of nurturance and support, there is a climate of restriction, demands and threats which frustrates growth and legitimate freedom of movement. Often, one or the other partner tries to resist this frustration through the sexual acting out of anger. This only confirms the other's fears and negative self-imagery, while setting-up a type of self-fulfilling prophecy situation.

If the relationship ends, usually with vindictive rage and destructive behaviour, both partners emerge scarred emotionally and even less capable of loving than before. The result is often reinforcement of a preference for casual, anonymous, even unsafe sexual encounters. The extent to which such motives of high-risk sexual behaviour are taken into account by health educators is a moot question!

Monogamy versus Promiscuity

It is perhaps a truism that insecurity breeds promiscuity. However, other powerful emotional factors are involved here too. An exclusive preference for promiscuity is in fact a form of compulsion, in spite of rationalization of it as an expression of 'liberation'. In asserting this, I am expressing a personal opinion which may be unpopular with certain activists. What follows is a brief analysis of how I perceive its origins, with a view to opening up pathways to commitment and the enrichment of relationships. Again, many of the issues are relevant, I believe, to heterosexual as well as to homosexual persons.

Many people, irrespective of sexual preference, would admit periods of promiscuity, either between relationships or in the process of coming to terms with their sexuality and exploring ways of expressing intimacy and affection. Sexual behaviour is often used as an antidote to grief or depression or as a way of acting out rage or anger. Sometimes it represents an unconscious attempt to find a lost love-object or a more satisfying partner. It is a common pattern among homosexual men in the era of AIDS when so many are facing multiple losses, or bereavement overload.

However, it is vital *not* to judge ourselves or others, but to try to understand such behaviour. This is the pathway to healing and growth! Freud and others have shown that much sexual behaviour is *not* a result of moral depravity. It flows rather from buried or largely unconscious sources. True freedom of choice can only evolve in the wake of insight.

The awakening of a capacity for mature, loving and stable, commited or monogamous relationships, sometimes requires professional help, especially necessary at times of grieving or when coping with the impact of exposure to HIV. Monogamy itself can never exist in the context of demands or threats. As an option, it is a freely offered gift and one expression of wholeness and the acquired art of loving.

The Art of Loving

Erich Fromm has provided a lucid analysis of what he refers to as a capacity for 'productive loving'. According to Fromm, loving is not an act, but an *art*, flowing from attitudes of mutual care, responsibility, respect and knowledge. It is above all an *intentional* emotion. It is marked by a relative absence of irrational fear, illusion and projection onto others of negative qualities (such as homophobia). The self-obsession and insecurity of immature relationships are replaced by a realistic concern for the unfolding mystery of another person, perceived in terms of actual qualities and needs. The loved person is no longer made a screen onto which the lover projects his or her own unresolved conflicts and infantile needs, not really perceiving the other very much at all!

Productive, mature love is both a stimulus to growth and a source of the deepest spiritual, peak experiences, as well as humor, fun, joy and well-being. It is marked by the expression of positive identity, rather than restriction, possessiveness and arrested growth.

Two people in a mature love relationship reach out from the emotional safety of their bonding to others, individuals or society, in recognition that their fullest growth as persons means contributing to a larger whole. Commitment is based upon shared intimacy, meaning, values and the awareness that sexuality itself is an expression of mutual affirmation, affection and spirituality. Others are included and supported, not regarded as rivals or shut out due to neurotic fears. Neither partner feels like a hostage with little or no freedom of movement.

In this context, monogamy may become an aspect of commitment and shared values. When it occurs, it is the exchange of a gift, offered in freedom, not in response to demands or as a concession to moralists or from a fear of HIV infection.

The transformation which makes this possible, however, often entails the prior overcoming of difficulties with sexual identity, intimacy and trust. Resolution of these issues may require professional help.

Relationship Counseling and Therapy

Participation in groups focusing upon personal growth and consciousness-raising is probably the most effective means of overcoming these obstacles to commitment and enrichment of relationships.

Typically, in such groups, memories, feelings and conflicts which have blocked previous attempts at bonding are relived in relation to group members in a non-judgemental setting of support, understanding and compassion. Unresolved issues concerning sexual identity, trust, intimacy and loss are addressed anew.

Group members rebuild poor self-images and gradually become capable of touching and being touched emotionally and of being genuinely expressive. Inward-turning anger and self-hatred are reversed. Resentment is replaced with forgiveness, fear with courage, cynicism with values, spiritual bankruptcy with a re-awakened awareness of meaning, of love for others, even for God, in whatever form the person understands God.

The 'miracle'—and it can seem a miracle—achieved as a result of this group process is painful and takes time, but it is a necessary condition for growth and change and, above all, for health, integration and wholeness. Part of the miracle, working on a collective level, might well be a genuine renaissance of commitment, accompanied by a rippling effect, whereby the capacity for loving in individuals spreads to entire communities.

Traditionally, homosexual relationships have lacked social support and legitimization. One task that homosexual and lesbian people face is the development of their own models of relating as well as value systems supportive of growth and commitment in their relationships. This is one challenge, at a collective level, linked to the presence of AIDS. Yet the issue of how to enrich relationships is also one confronting the dominant society, bereft as it is becoming of traditional spiritual values and guidelines.

PART FOUR

PSYCHOTHERAPY COUNSELING AND PASTORAL CARE: ACTIVITIES AND EXERCISES

CHAPTER ELEVEN

Relaxation, Visualization, Meditation and Reflections for Discussion

The two chapters in Part Four are intended primarily for the practical use of therapists, counsellors, clergypersons and group facilitators who work in the HIV/AIDS field and with people facing life-threatening illnesses generally.

In this chapter we examine first the techniques of relaxation and meditation. The value of these techniques is discussed in chapter seven (see pages 52–55).

What follows then are a number of reflections on such significant issues such as social oppression, stigma, mortality, homosexual identity, emotional responses to HIV/AIDS and spirituality in infected persons and their significant others—partners and families.

These reflections can be used for individual study, but are more useful as prompts to discussion of the issues raised, within the group therapy situation or in workshops for counselors, therapists and other workers.

At an appropriate moment during a group session one of the reflections may be presented orally or played from a pre-recorded audio tape. The members of the group can then be invited to discuss the issues raised.

Relaxation

INTRODUCTION

Progressive muscle relaxation is valuable in itself as a means of reducing stress and anxiety and is used for this purpose by many behaviour therapists. I describe its use here as a preparation for visualization or guided imagery exercises, aiming to help patients get in touch with their emotions and with deeper aspects of self or personal identity.

The content of the visualizations themselves should, ideally, reflect the issues surfacing in psychotherapy or counselling at particular stages of work with patients. This is consistent with the goal of using these techniques as adjuncts to psychotherapy or counselling. Patients may be asked to practice these exercises regularly for periods of fifteen minutes or more between formal sessions. Some health professionals record relaxation instructions and visualizations on audiotapes for the use of their patients.

INSTRUCTIONS FOR RELAXATION

Patients are asked to ensure periods of about thirty minutes when they will be free of distraction or interruption from others or the telephone. I generally suggest that they recline on a bed or sit in a comfortable chair, having placed on some suitable music. Certain baroque passages, for example the Pachelbel Canon in D and selections from Bach, Handel and Albinoni and Gregorian Chant or other pieces that are gentle and slow-moving help to induce relaxation and trance-like states. The preliminary relaxation instructions are as follows and are to be spoken in a slow, calm manner, pausing to allow participants to act on the instructions.

'Allow yourself to drift slowly away with the music. Focus first on your feet. Note any sensations or feelings that are there—tension, soreness, lightness or heaviness. Now relax your toes, then your feet, letting go of any tension. As your muscles relax, breathe in and out, freely and deeply, continuing to listen to my voice and to drift further away with the music.

'Focus now on your calf muscles. Again note any feelings that are there and as you relax the muscles, let go of any tension, breathing freely and deeply, in and out. Relax your thighs, your buttocks, breathing in and out, freely and deeply.

'Focus now on your pelvis—your midsection. Note any feelings of tightness. Relax the muscles, letting go of the tightness or tension. Continue to drift away with the music. Now relax your back and shoulders. As you breathe freely and deeply, relax your diaphragm and chest muscles.

'Focus upon your hands. Note any feelings of numbness or tingling, lightness or heaviness. Now relax your fingers, then your hands, breathing in and out, freely and deeply. Relax your forearms, upper arms, biceps, triceps. As you become more and more wrapped-up in the music and drift away, further and further, relax your neck muscles, letting go of any feelings of tension. Now, relax your forehead, scalp, then your jaw.

'Note your eyelids, and as you relax they become heavier and heavier. You are beginning to feel heavy, drowsy and sleepy. Just drift along with the music, as far away as you like.

'In a moment, I shall count from one to ten and as I do, you will become more and more drowsy and sleepy. As I count, you might imagine that you are in a slowly descending lift. ONE, beginning to move downwards into sleep; TWO, THREE, deeper and deeper; FOUR, still moving downwards; FIVE, heavier and heavier; SIX, more and more sleepy; SEVEN, EIGHT, deeper and deeper; NINE, TEN; deeply relaxed, drowsy and sleepy.

'Allow yourself to drift away for a few moments longer, with the music. Then we shall begin with the first visualization exercise'. (Or with a reflection.) Alternative methods of inducing relaxation and altered states of consciousness in preparation for visualization, include breathing exercises which involve focusing upon the movement and passage of the breath from its beginning to end and the use of visual stimuli such as lighted tapers which can help focus attention.

Some Examples of Creative Visualization

Again, speak these in a slow, calm way, allowing time for participants to focus on each new development of the image.

CLEANSING WATER

'Allow the music to become like a pure, crystal-clear stream of sound, flowing like water, in and through your mind, gently cleansing, washing away all fear and negativity.

'Just allow this lovely stream to become a kind of sacred spring, absolving, dissolving away feelings of guilt, shame and any sense you may have of being isolated or trapped. Perhaps you will begin to sense a lightness and relief, as heavy burdens and feelings are washed away by the flowing stream.'

HEALING LIGHT

'Now, try to allow the music to become a softly dawning light or an inner radiance, slowly rising, glowing, in your mind's eye, like a sun, dispelling darkness and gloomy feelings.

'Perhaps as this happens, you will begin to sense and feel something like a shimmering light, flooding in through the windows of your mind... streaming in and through your soul, your consciousness. Allow this inner light to form ripples of joy, waves of delight, passing across your mind, into and through your body.

'The ripples and waves of light and feeling may be like those formed by a pebble dropping into a pond.

'Just allow whatever lovely sensations and feelings are appearing to fill your mind, dispelling inner gloom and emptiness.'

HOLDING PRESENCE

'As you attend and become more and more responsive to the music, allow it to lift you up, to carry and transport you to some lofty mountain top or peak in your imagination or mind's eye. Perhaps you will find yourself in a space of unexpectedly clear vision, after your ascent to the peak of the mountain. Spend a moment looking around you.

'You may gradually begin to experience some images, faces or perhaps a Presence and a growing sense of closeness and proximity to whoever this Presence is as it becomes more clear to you.

'Just allow whatever is now starting to happen in your mind to surface, to reveal itself, as you experience more of the stillness and light of your mountain top or peak awareness.

'As you let go, surrendering more and more to whatever is happening, you may experience a sense of being held, cared for, accepted as you are, right now at this moment, by the figure or Presence which has appeared in your consciousness.

'Allow yourself to be held, strengthened and empowered. Perhaps, through this holding, you will also experience something of a loving energy. If so, direct this energy to those parts of yourself which are most in need of healing.'

COMMENT

Creative visualizations such as these are useful in awakening active, positive emotions and mood-states. They are used after the induction of deep relaxation or hypnosis. Suggestions useful for bringing people back to normal consciousness include counting from 10 back to 1, with instruction to return fully to the room, with perhaps a comment about possible rippling effects of pleasant emotions, carrying over into the waking-state.

Meditation

Along the way of the pilgrimage to healing regular meditation helps to expand and to deepen consciousness of the (unconscious) psyche, self and God-image within the person. Deep meditation creates states of stillness and 'peak experiences' of joy, elation, energy and vitality. Visions or images of an inner light (for example the sun or a flame) are quite common.

Moreover, empirical research has linked meditation to enhanced quality of life and increased survival time in cancer patients. Recent data and my own clinical observations suggest that such findings will probably also hold for people living with HIV/AIDS (see Solomon, 1987). However, further research is necessary to elucidate the effects of meditation upon both immunity and the progression of illness in HIV antibody positive persons.

Meditation is a spiritual discipline, which can involve the use of breathing exercises, mantras, chanting and certain forms of imagery, including icons, to awaken experiences of the deeper self or God-presence within the person. Meditation is best learned from a reputable, experienced teacher—many health professionals, religious or clergy have appropriate training.

One type, Siddha meditation, associated with the name of Gurumayi, is widely taught and its effects upon immunity, survival-time and quality of life in cancer patients are currently being evaluated by Magarey and others.

Two practical introductory texts on meditation, written within a Christian framework, are *Moment of Christ*, by Benedictine monk John Main, and *The Marriage of East and West* by another Benedictine, living in India, Bede Griffiths. Books describing meditation techniques can be valuable, but in my opinion personal instruction and experience are more effective than reading alone.

As a spiritual discipline, meditation transcends both traditional religious and denominational boundaries. Such divisions, I believe, have their origins in human egos and reflect little, if anything, of that living, authentic experience, the 'knowing' of God, described by the saints and mystics of all ages, for example by Hildegaard of Bingen, Teresa of Avila, and John of the Cross in the west.

Meditation touches those deeper dimensions of the human psyche which Carl Jung describes as 'archetypal', that is, universal and timeless. Those who do experience something of the deeper self know that God is infinitely greater than the narrow images and even the most esoteric theologies which humankind has created.

It is quite possible that the spiritual awakening which meditation aims to facilitate can help Christians recover the meaning of their rich store of religious symbols and sacraments. Meditation assists at the marriage of head and heart, intellect and feeling and it helps to establish a true correspondence between the outward sense and visible sign of ritual and sacrament and the real, inner process of psychic transformation. I shall illustrate this vital point in chapter thirteen with a series of practical, spiritual exercises, using certain traditional Christian religious symbols.

Finally, meditation might well be one powerful way of providing an injection of spirituality into western medicine, to help heal its 'dis-ease' with the mental and spiritual dimensions of life-threatening illness, such as cancer and HIV/AIDS.

Meditation teaches us that if we truly open ourselves up to the experience of the unconscious, unknown, deeper self or God-image within us, then God does not withold himself from us. It is a matter of surrendering the ego, with an attitude of humility, as we practice such spiritual disciplines. The experiences themselves are simply gifts of grace—of unconditional love.

Some religious patients use the images which come to them during meditation or visualization during their medical treatment, for example, being 'transfused' by the blood of Christ or 'filled' with the fire of the Holy Spirit in chemotherapy. This is perhaps a wonderfully enlightened form of holism in therapy, expressing an inner sense and experience of the marriage of the human and the divine. On a more personal level, I have discovered through meditation something of what it means to experience oneself as a kind of lens, the function of which is to magnify and to project into the world a source of light, loving and healing energy, infinitely greater than one's ego. This is an experience of oneself, paradoxically, as being both nothing and everything!

Reflections for Group Discussion

'ECCE HOMO!': BEHOLD THE MAN!

Imagine, just for a few moments, that you are to be personally present at an event or happening which truly seems to represent a turning point or crossroads in human evolution and history. For in fact you may be about to find yourself actually taking part, in your imagination, in a kind of 'transition' experience. Time and eternity may seem to intersect—somehow crossing for an instant—in the stillness of your minds, much as a searchlight pierces the darkness across the night sky.

Allow yourself to be present at this event, *just as you are now*: happy or sad, calm or tense, resentful or loving, spiritual or passionately sceptical, about anything divine or Godlike, about yourself and humanity in general. Just *be who you are*, right now, at this moment in time.

Perhaps too you are present only out of curiosity or because you are a part of a crowd; bored, having little else to do but to watch another execution for the crime of sedition. This particular criminal is said to be a little 'strange': he tried to stir up protest or insurrection among the social misfits, outcasts and moral lepers in this city. He even commited sacrilege in the precints of the Temple by creating a disturbance—by disrupting a very profitable business run to fill the coffers of the religious establishment.

It is the crucifixion of Christ! Capture the surroundings as the drama begins to unfold in your imagination. It is a very hot, oppressive afternoon. A slowly sinking sun is reflected in the gathering storm clouds. An uncanny twilight seems to be descending upon the crowd with its murmuring, babbling voices—and the stench of sweat!

Behold the man! He is stretched . . . suspended high . . . in the strange twilight . . . nailed and tied to rough wooden beams . . . his sweat mingles with dust and the blood flowing from his face, hands and feet. He wears a crown of thorns, a mocking parody of his odd claims and pretensions—not the sort of king or leader expected or wanted these days by the establishment! He fights for air, screams out from his inner void, God-forsaken. The struggle continues on the cross.

Behold the man! He is stripped bare, exposed, uncovered, naked, bereft of everything—of all status, power, pretence. His body is broken, fragile, in the hands of oppression and cruelty. His body bears the weight and the outward visible marks of stigma and shame—of flagellation—at the hands of human bigotry, fear, hatred and indifference. He is held up to public ridicule and left to die—as will be the countless victims and scapegoats of humanity's collective Shadow throughout all of human history. The struggle continues on the cross!

Now, look into his eyes! Is he insane? Is he just another deluded, crazy troublemaker or would-be prophet? Apparently, he claimed to be the Son of God, so that the high priest tore off his own garments, in the early hours of this morning. For this, the man hangs now, in the descending darkness, suspended between time and eternity—in 'transition', letting go gradually, saying something to his mother and closest companion. The struggle continues on the cross!

Look again into his eye! The eyes of the man who was not what was wanted or expected in a Messiah and who refused the lure and temptation of worldly political power and triumph over others, even the Romans. What do you sense in his eyes? In the face of the man whose vision, presence and compassion seemed to penetrate so deeply into the Shadow or hell of human destructiveness, suffering and 'dis-ease'—touching, healing and transforming. He descended into hell; into the darkest moments and places of human history, even here and now.

The storm bursts . . . lightning flashes and illuminates the man. The earth seems to resound . . . to convulse. He is stretched, dismembered almost, suspended now in his dying moment of surrender, letting go of the human ego, completing, realizing the destiny he feared, the purpose and the meaning he asked to be spared as he sweated blood, terrified, in the garden. He cries out for the last time. His ego has surrendered to the myth which motivated his life. It is consummated . . . over . . . finished! Eternal!

But the struggle continues on the cross . . . throughout history. In the timeless endless faces of human suffering . . . in the many faces of oppression . . . in Auschwitz and Chile . . . in the faces of those sick, dying and stigmatized, because of HIV . . . yet outcast, abandoned by those within the church, who wash their hands, in righteousness, while others, cast lots for political power, prestige or for a Nobel Prize.

For whom or for what meaning, purpose or value would you, personally be prepared, symbolically speaking, to go to the cross, to give your life? What is your personal myth, mission or unfinished business in the world?

HOMOSEXUALITY AND THE 'NATURAL LAW'

Social and moral, as well as theological attitudes towards homosexuality have traditionally reflected pre-scientific views of human sexuality. In particular, the 'Natural Law' argument, stated by the medieval theologian, Thomas Aquinas, has exerted a powerful influence in shaping the thinking of the western church and of society generally. It still does.

Aquinas was writing in an age whose collective consciousness was still possessed by the spirit of the Greek philosopher Aristotle, and two centuries before the rise of empirical science. What, in essence, was his argument?

Briefly, Aquinas argued that all acts which are due to free will and also contrary to the revealed natural order, the design or creation of God, are of necessity sinful or immoral. Thus, if the 'homosexual condition' itself and the overt expression of homosexual impulses are freely chosen and are also contrary to the divine design of human sexuality, which exists solely for the purpose of procreation, then both of these things are seriously sinful.

The natural law argument, whether or not it is buttressed or propped up with selected scriptural quotations, is seriously flawed and erroneous, on both logical and factual scientific grounds. Further, Aquinas could not have foreseen that the social effects of his argument would include the oppression, stigmatization, suffering and death of numberless souls!

The scientific truth is, of course, that the homosexual condition is *not* freely chosen at all; rather it is discovered. It is in fact an intrinsic part of the being, creation and personal identity of homosexual individuals. The discovery of one's homosexual identity is, in principle, the same as the discovery of a heterosexual identity in others, except for the context in which this self-revelation occurs. Prior to the discovery of their sexual identity, homosexual people have already internalized the negativity, fear, hatred and stigmatization of the dominant culture or society. They have internalized homophobia.

They thus begin to fear, to cover-up, to hate and to feel bad or ashamed, of this vital part of their inner selves. They may become self-destructive, and so vulnerable to HIV. Once they are infected, they are at risk for an early death, from this and many other causes.

If such homosexual people, experiencing inner 'dis-ease' with their sexuality, have not yet been damaged beyond repair, they may seek professional help from a minister, priest, counselor or psychotherapist. They may or may not be fortunate in their reaching out and choice of a helping person.

If they are lucky, they will discover the truth, they will experience an 'enlightenment' into the deeper self and into their homosexuality. They will be cleansed, in therapy, of the burden of fear, shame and resentment and will be absolved of the need of pretending not to feel what they do feel and of feeling what they do not feel at all.

They will experience a revelation of their essential humanness, of their similarity to others. For them, as for all of us, the real question is now not who I love, man or woman, but *that* I love and have become truly capable of loving myself and others.

One compelling answer to the Natural Law argument, which continues to buttress moralistic and homophobic attitudes, is essentially quite simple.

The nature and quality of human love, insofar as it embraces the whole person—psyche or soul, as well as the body—cannot be defined by or confined to particular anatomical regions and appendages. To claim otherwise is to confuse both Eros and Agape (spiritual love, empathy, compassion) with Sexus—the purely physical, bodily expression of lust, as well as genuine love.

The actual experience of love in its wholeness is its own justification and validation—its own beauty, truth and goodness. Such an experience cannot, of its very nature, be confined to or identified with acts whose sole purpose is procreation—as if love itself is a mere 'accident', a by-product of the reproductive intention or aim! That is to say, love is of the substance of the human psyche, it is not an accidental accretion to purely sexual, reproductive acts.

The Natural Law position requires unnatural mental gymnastics and twists of logic, as well as the denial of experiential and scientific facts. Ultimately, it is pernicious in its effects and destructive of love itself—insofar as it degrades human beings to the status of beast (as if devoid of soul) whose sexuality is designed only to fulfill reproductive ends or purposes.

This argument then, denies specifically the obvious fact that humans, unlike other animals, experience sexuality as an instrument or pathway for the expression of love, as a substantial mental and spiritual dimension of their very being.

It matters not what anatomical regions become the objects or receptacles of one's bodily passions. Rather, what matters is the attitude and presence, the *disposition* of love, as the motivation of one's acts. The presence of genuine love is the essence and spring of real morality and it is of God—a fact understood and grasped by the mystics.

Christian fundamentalists still tend to cling to the argument that the homosexual condition itself reflects the disorder existing in the world because of the fall of humanity described in the Old Testament Book of Genesis. The argument, however, is fundamentally flawed and erroneous. It represents a further example of that literalism in interpreting scripture which also denies scientific revelations about the evolution and structure of the universe, as well as human sexuality.

Ultimately, biblical revelation and empirical science cannot be mutually contradictory. And yet religious fundamentalists are typically terrified of the ambiguities and complexities of the world and of human nature, as these are illuminated by empirical science.

They therefore resemble the theologians of Galileo's day who refused to look through telescopes out of fear of discovering material facts that might have challenged or threatened their narrow beliefs and limited views of the world. It is as if their image of God is far too small!

In reality, the many faces and variations of human sexual response, orientation, object-relationship and love all seem to reflect the intrinsic nature of an evolutionary process. The sheer complexity and elegance of this process is awesome and magnificent. For it appears that life and human reflective-consciousness have emerged from transformations in matter, whereby more and more complex and improbable arrangements of elementary particles create higher and higher forms of order. Evolution then, in one sense, is a movement from randomness or chaos towards order—the reverse of the situation envisioned by the fundamentalists.

At the summit of humanity's gradual evolutionary ascent the brain has become the organ both of human reflective-consciousness and of a remarkable creativity, flexibility and capacity, even for contemplation of the imprint of the divine upon the psyche or soul. Our religious symbols appear or are revealed, on this mountain of 'transfiguration', in consciousness. The diversity of sexual orientation, attachment and bonding processes mirrors and expresses what is known of our evolutionary origins.

As both created being and creator, each human person is destined to participate in God, in evolution, on a cultural plane and in the extension of the incarnation through historic time. One dimension of the pilgrimage to healing for each person is his or her discovery of a unique meaning, role or 'personal myth' in such a wonderful, awesome order, design and creative process as it is!

OPPRESSION, STIGMA AND THE KILLING PROCESS

HIV is an insidious and lethal 'presence', casting its grim shadow over the lives of millions of people globally. HIV is superbly equipped, in its evolution, for its function of destroying the individual's biological defence system, that is, the body's immunity.

However, HIV has found powerful and co-operative allies in those dark 'principalities and powers' known and materialized in the many forms and faces of social oppression and stigma. These sinister forces masquerade also in the guise of prejudice, fear, hatred and homophobic attitudes towards those who are different because of their sexual and affectional preference.

Thus, by some strange coincidence, HIV seems to have selectively targeted persons who belong to what is, perhaps, the most despised, stigmatized, feared, hated and persecuted minority group in all of human history. Why them? Why us? Why me? Is there no redemption, liberation or end to it all?

So, what about the killing? It is now occurring on a scale, which is far beyond the dreams of history's most notorious architects of genocide. Could the killings somehow be linked with that mass crucifixion of souls, carried out in the name of oppression, bigotry and prejudice—mass scape-goating of 'sacrificial victims'?

Do powerful psychic forces exist, which cause many people to be especially vulnerable to HIV, once infected or exposed? How could oppression kill—softly, subtly, but certainly?

Oppression, stigma, homophobia and other damaging attitudes are taken into the unconscious psyche through the most vulnerable and significant periods in the individual's personality and identity formation. This subtle, insidious process of internalization of negativity has begun even before the discovery that the person's sexuality and other parts of the inner self are different.

It occurs largely through parents and other symbolically significant figures, who act as unconscious channels of social values, norms and prejudices. How, then, is the imprint of such powerful, negative, damaging forces upon the unconscious mind to be identified and recognized? How might internalized oppression, stigma, homophobia and negativity impact upon immunity and the outcome of HIV infection?

First, let us consider what happens to the person on a mental and spiritual plane. What is the imprint of oppressive, devaluing, invalidating and belittling attitudes upon the soul? The following pattern of factors can usually be observed:

a) repressed anger and rage;

b) denied, disowned, split-off or incompletely accepted homosexual identity, with underlying guilt and shame;

c) proneness to self-hatred, depression and suicidism;

d) poor self esteem, negative identity, playing out the 'victim' role;

e) social withdrawal, isolation and loneliness;

f) lack of a positive sense of meaning, purpose and direction in life.

Some of you may have noticed a remarkable coincidence between this profile and something else. This something else is, of course, the pattern of psychological factors which scientific research has linked with immunosuppression and with the progression of AIDS-related disease. The story with cancer is very similar and we must add to the factors just mentioned the link between loss through death or separation and immune-suppression.

What is to be done? How can psychospiritual methods of therapy help to exorcise the destructive, damaging effects of oppression and stigma and, perhaps, arrest the 'killing' process? How do we fight against and overcome these allies of HIV, through our work together in this group?

Consider what happens after diagnosis of HIV antibody positive status. Beyond the stages of coping with loss described by Elisabeth Kübler-Ross—shock, disbelief, denial, anger, bargaining, depression and so on—patients usually experience what is known as an emotional 'regression.' This is essentially a state of enhanced vulnerability, dependency and helplessness, which occurs as patients begin to confront the frightening implications of the diagnosis.

Powerful memories and feelings are re-awakened. Rage, anger and depression about past experiences of loss and disappointment, as well as buried or unresolved issues about gay identity or 'coming out', re-surface at this time. So also does much 'unfinished business' with partners and families. Anger and rage are often dumped or displaced onto lovers and other significant persons.

Suicidal behaviour, both serious attempts and gestures, reflect not only despair or hopelessness but also the acting out of repressed or unconscious anger towards others, in the past as well the present. More serious suicide attempts can sometimes be understood as acts of unconscious 'homicide'. By killing the self, the patient is also destroying all of the mental images, memories and emotions that are within.

Group support, and especially the therapeutic expression of intense and scary emotions such as rage, reduce the risk of suicide and of other self-destructive behaviour like alcohol or drug abuse. (Some doctors, unfortunately, in issuing prescriptions for drugs like Rohypnol to HIV antibody positive patients, may be handing out death warrants.) It is well known that substance abuse can become a passive or indirect expression of suicidal impulses as well as being immuno-suppressive.

The diagnosis of HIV antibody positive status usually results in a re-awakening or re-surfacing of unresolved issues about loss, disappointment, sexual identity, stigmatization and basic trust. Many patients, at this stage, describe themselves as somehow 'damaged', 'unclean' or 'leprous' and as wanting to isolate, to hide away or to become invisible. The underlying emotions tend to be shame, embarrassment, guilt and worthlessness. The present is generally misperceived, in terms of the past.

A vital part of group psychotherapy is the uncovering, working through and resolution of such underlying or unconscious issues, memories and feelings. Such deep interventions should be attempted only by properly trained therapists who can provide the necessary experiences of holding, handling and containment, interpreting rather than personalizing patients' emotional responses.

Holding, handling, containment, empathy and compassion are essential if the patient needs to experience, to acknowledge and to express repressed anger, rage, despair and depression. Getting rid of such underlying negativity and destructiveness is only possible as people become less guarded or defensive in a context or situation of safety and trust.

During the group work, 'repressed' and inward-turning anger or self-hatred are reversed as buried feelings are expressed and negative self images reappraised. People slowly become more self-accepting, discovering new positive, creative parts of themselves. They learn to forgive themselves and others—to receive and to give unconditional love—perhaps for the first time. The result is enhanced *self esteem* and enrichment of personal relationships.

Through the group work, the inner sense of powerlessness and helplessness or dependency are replaced with a boosted sense of real personal power and control over one's own health and that of others. This change occurs through commitment to the group process and as a result of active participation in other health-enhancing activities, such as exercise and meditation.

On a spiritual plane, as members of the group, patients may experience their participation as a powerful means or pathway to a deeper sense of self worth, validation and meaning in life. This occurs partly through a deepening awareness of belonging and communion in a collective growth and healing process.

As members of the living body of the group, each person has a unique function, gifts and contribution to make to others and to the whole body, which the group represents. And the group as a whole can become a powerful force whose fighting spirit is mobilized against oppression, stigma and killing.

DENIAL: ITS MANY FACES

Denial is a primitive, defensive response to perceived threat both within the individual psyche or consciousness and in the external world of objective facts. As a mental defense mechanism, it is a process of refusing to look and of turning away from perceptions, ideas, impulses and feelings which would cause intense fear or anxiety if they were consciously acknowledged or attended to.

Denial is an almost universal initial response to disaster and to such life threatening situations as the diagnosis of cancer or of positive HIV antibody status. Elisabeth Kübler-Ross, in such books as *On Death and Dying* and *AIDS: The Ultimate Challenge*, describes denial as the first of several stages in the process of grieving and of coping with death and loss.

Denial defends or protects the individual—temporarily—against being overwhelmed by such powerful emotions as terror, preventing the experience of being frozen with fear or paralyzed. It is as if the danger or threat, once denied or even not yet acknowledged, does not exist or has disappeared magically through wishful fantasy.

Denial presents many faces which are nevertheless quite easy to recognize, especially as it is linked with the behaviour patterns of avoidance and flight. Let us consider some of the ways in which denial avoidance and taking-flight are revealed in response to the growing presence of HIV/AIDS in the community.

One way is certainly the powerful resistance which exists to screening for HIV antibody status in high-risk groups—especially given the knowledge that early diagnosis can lead to effective medical and psychological interventions.

The denial is expressed in such commonly-heard statements as 'It can't happen to me', 'I'd rather not know about it', 'I couldn't be infected because I have sex only with healthy looking partners', or 'I feel indestructible, so my daily use of drugs and alcohol isn't going to affect my health or T-cells.' Other fairly obvious examples include turning or running away from people with symptoms of AIDS because they represent 'mirrors' and reminders of illness and death, and engaging in *known* high risk practices for the transmission of HIV, such as unsafe sex and needle-sharing. Attempts to pass as straight, and other covering-up strategies during the coming-out process in gay men, usually reflect at least a partial denial, as well as a disowning or splitting-off, of this part of the inner self or personality.

On a social or collective level, it is very probable that the 'Grim Reaper' commercials, shown on Australian television a few years ago and based on fear as a motivating force, would have strongly reinforced the tendency to use denial as a defense mechanism, especially for members of high risk groups. These graphic commercials, with their images of death and destruction, aroused high levels of fear about AIDS, without suggesting immediate, constructive ways of reducing anxiety or of coping with threat, particularly for people in high risk groups or, worse, already infected with HIV.

It is also likely that homophobic attitudes would have been intensified by such media messages, resulting in an increased tendency towards the targeting and victimization of people perceived as belonging to high risk groups. Scapegoating is one example of the social use of the mechanism of 'attack-as-defence', against a real or imagined threat.

Kübler-Ross and many others have pointed out that our culture is a 'death-denying' one. However, this pervasive attitude tends in itself to block the adoption of truly 'death-defying', self-nurturing and constructive actions and behaviour patterns, vital both to individual survival and to a society living with HIV/AIDS. No community or subculture can survive unless its individual members survive.

Denial is a huge problem because it precludes or inhibits patterns of behaviour which lead to effective mastery and control of HIV's lethal presence in our midst. For many people, the retrovirus is no longer merely an external threat that can be overlooked or avoided; it is already present within them.

Somehow, denial must be replaced by a realistic acknowledgement of the situation, followed by death-defiance and a genuine fighting spirit, if HIV is ultimately to be challenged and overcome. How can such a process occur and be facilitated?

Sometimes, denial passes spontaneously. This may occur through the onset of obvious symptoms of HIV infection or through the loss of a lover or friend. Under such circumstances, denial is more difficult to sustain. However, letting go of denial can be facilitated in other, more positive ways.

For a start, media messages should aim to eliminate or to minimize fear and stigma, while emphasizing the constructive steps people can take to resolve anxiety. Practical ways of regaining personal power, control and responsibility for one's own health should be promoted instead of attitudes of pessimism and of hopelessness about HIV. The dissemination of information about the benefits of early diagnosis, medical and psychological treatments could make the process of actually facing the realities of HIV/AIDS much easier.

As denial begins to recede, it becomes possible, with skilled counseling and psychotherapy, to work with the real issues, which have been overlooked, covered up or avoided. These issues include all of the personality, stress and emotional factors which are likely, according to scientific research, to influence immunity and the disease progression in HIV antibody positive people.

REPRESSION AND MORALITY

Many of the revolutionary insights into the human psyche generated by such visionaries as Sigmund Freud and Carl Jung have yet to filter into society's collective consciousness. Western society still tends to cling to the illusion—or delusion—of possessing a rational enlightenment into itself, as well as grasping the lawfulness of the material cosmos in which it is embodied.

Illumination into the inner self and of the dynamic forces at work in the unconscious psyche eludes all but a tiny minority of a supposedly civilized, educated society. Aside from the epidemics of madness and genocide unleashed at various times, humanity seems to be in search of a soul and thus easy prey to various cults, sects and fanatical religious movements. Even human sexuality seems all too often to be a problem or source of 'dis-ease'.

In the era of HIV/AIDS, primitive and powerful irrational psychic forces seem to be manifested in patterns of homophobic, oppressive stigmatization and backlash, often facilitated and encouraged by religious fundamentalists. Such attitudes and behaviour, together with the tendency within western Christianity to negate or to repress human bodiliness, sensuality and feeling, while overvaluing the purely rational, point to the presence of a potentially dangerous or even fatal imbalance in the psyche. It may not be purely a coincidence that this very imbalance seems to be mirrored, in an enhanced vulnerability to HIV itself, in infected persons.

This repression and imbalance and the consequent splitting in the psyche seems to be directly reflected in the mentality of certain people who could be best described as 'moral pygmies.' Such individuals often inhabit ecclesiastical structures, adopting a defensive posture of judgement, while lacking genuine understanding, care and compassion towards those who are living with HIV/AIDS.

What is the nature of the repression to which I am referring, and what do its consequences seem to be, both individually and collectively? Put simply, repression is a mental defence mechanism, operating so as to exclude or to banish from consciousness, ideas, perceptions, impulses, memories and feelings which would cause distress or pain if allowed into awareness. Repression, then, works to avoid the awakening of emotional pain, which comes through the remembering or re-presentation of unconscious contents or material in consciousness.

However, although the defense of repression, and its

more primitive cousin denial, act so as to maintain emotional equilibrium or a rather illusory peace of mind, the cost to the individual's mental economy is enormous. Considerable energy is consumed in a constant struggle to keep threatening material out of consciousness, almost as if the person is in a chronic state of vigilance, self-watching or censorship.

Repressed content, simply by being made 'unconscious', does not, of course, cease to exist. It always reappears in disguised form, for example, in dreams, slips of the tongue, unexplained moods, neurotic symptoms and psychosomatic disorders, like migraine headaches or duodenal ulcers. Freud himself referred to this process as 'the return of the repressed.' Repression usually results in a gross impoverishment of the personality, so that in severe cases one is reminded of the image of a withered tree—devoid of animation and passion, bored and boring—lifeless!

Repression is frequently, if not always linked also with projection; what remains buried or unconscious, is perceived and reacted to as if it now existed, outside, in the external world or in others. Thus, for example, repression of the Shadow is followed by the discovery of its qualities embodied in someone else, or in some minority group, who can then be attacked with righteous indignation or demonic fury. It is very much a matter of criticising the speck in one's brother's eye, while overlooking the beam in one's own!

Repression and projection are powerful forces at work, through the dynamics of scapegoating and social prejudice, whether directed towards racial minorities or gays or those with HIV/AIDS.

These brief reflections upon the nature and consequences of repression may help to clarify certain difficult issues of human morality and spirituality, especially as these apply to homosexuality and AIDS. First, in a state of repression genuine moral and ethical choice are, in fact, quite impossible. It is simply not possible to take a stand or to make enlightened choices about parts or dimensions of the inner self, which are neither known, nor possessed, fully.

Second, with regard to sexuality, those whose impulses and feelings are repressed or who are acting compulsively, because they are still unconscious of their motives are essentially in an amoral or pre-moral position, with limited freedom of choice. Only as sexuality and underlying motives become conscious and are fully owned are people capable of moral choice.

Once people's sexuality is truly their own, they are free to express or to renounce it according to their insight into the self and their values and beliefs. Insofar as they are now more conscious, whole, balanced and at one with themselves, they may now also be capable of authentic self-sacrifice, love and holiness. In a real sense, they are new creations, as the old patterns of defence, illusion and inner-splitting have passed away. They have experienced healing of the 'dis-ease' they had with themselves. The encounter with the Shadow is a necessary condition for the attainment of wholeness and for authenticity in human relationships, whether personal, professional or pastoral.

SEXUALITY AND THE SEARCH FOR TRANSCENDENCE

A particularly common symptom of the so-called 'mid-life crisis' or 'passage' experience is the emerging awareness of an apparent need for sexual adventures or excitement. This experience seems to possess an almost irresistable quality and it occurs in previously stable individuals with strong religious beliefs, as well as those whose patterns of bonding and human attachment have been either disappointing or dysfunctional.

The symptom of craving for new sexual adventures can be disturbing to previously stable personalities especially. It is as if they have been taken by surprise, caught unprepared and quite unconscious of what is befalling them, or seeming to possess them from within. And the experience does happen, with a remarkable regularity, to such apparently unlikely people as clergy and happily-married professional and business persons.

This particular form of unexpected encounter with one of the many faces of the unconscious Shadow tends to throw the person off-balance. Often the individual's response is to greet the Shadow, in its manifestation of unruly passions, with a bad conscience, that is to say, with feelings of guilt and shame. The person may attempt to dissolve such painful emotions by turning to alcohol or drugs.

The problem seems to be that until the individual becomes more fully enlightened and deeply conscious of the powerful psychic forces or motives *behind* the craving for sexual adventure, he or she will tend to act *as if* the only real need is to fulfil the fantasies, dreams and desires, which are now revealed to and flooding into ego-consciousness. Moral judgements and counsel which seek simply to facilitate suppression are of little or no value to the person in this predicament.

The truly wise counselor or therapist knows that the patient is caught between the devil and the deep—that he or she faces a crucial dilemma in the life cycle. It may seem as if both acting and not acting upon the sexual feelings are equally perilous or dangerous for the patient. The therapist's role is, of course, to listen and above all to respect the patient's dilemma, in the knowledge that its origins are in a vital and as yet largely unconscious psychic movement or process which has a transformative significance.

Ultimately, this perceived need for new sexual adventures is not exclusively or even primarily about sexuality, but it reflects a deeper, unacknowledged quest or search. If people do act upon overtly sexual feelings, they can be helped to observe their responses and to explore whether in fact the experience does represent the manifestation of a deeper, largely unconscious issue or conflict, which now needs to be confronted on the inner pilgrimage towards healing, transformation and wholeness. One such question is what it means to be entering the autumn or second half of life, when the challenge is that of facing death and of finding an authentic sense of spirituality or meaning.

For many homosexual men, the issues of the second half of life are complicated by other unresolved conflicts and obstacles to individuation, personal growth or self-realization. One difficulty is that of grieving, of letting go of an image of self as the *puer aeternus* or eternal youth—very common in narcissistic personalities and reminiscent of the Dorian Gray myth, in which the portrait of the person became younger in appearance as the real individual aged more and more visibly. The youthful person, with whom the older man believes he has fallen in love, is a self-object or representation, that is to say, an idealized and eroticized mirror-image of the individual's lost youth or of the wounded-child part of the inner self.

Other homosexual persons enter the mid-life crisis or transition with the experience of an incomplete 'coming-out' process, associated with a need to integrate or to bring together their homosexual identity with both the feeling and spiritual sides of the inner self and personality, as a whole. With this process of integration within the psyche emerges the need to discover an authentic sense of identification with, belonging to and membership in a community, which supports and empowers the person's true self, and the fulfillment of his or her personal myth or sense of meaning in life.

The quest for sexual adventures, in mid-life or when facing the implications of HIV positive antibody status, can often be understood as unconscious attempts either to resist the letting go of past or changing self-images or to complete an arrested 'coming-out' process or to find an inner harmony, balance and wholeness, reflecting the marriage between sexuality and spirituality. The task in therapy is to facilitate the expansion and deepening of consciousness of such powerful, dynamic forces.

And sometimes those in this situation need to re-evaluate or even to let go of those self-images, beliefs and human attachments which create obstacles to the process of individuation, that is, to the fulfilment of their real goals, dreams and meanings. Such letting go implies loss, grief and pain which need to be acknowledged and worked through.

More generally, the perceived need or craving for sexual adventure conceals a cry or scream, deep within the soul, for meaning and self-transcendence. In other words, the individual is searching, unconsciously for a spiritual awakening, a conversion or transformation experience, not unlike those associated with the names of such persons as St Francis of Assisi, St Vincent de Paul or Matt Talbot. As Viktor Frankl has suggested, the apparent pursuit of sexual excitement represents an avoidance of or flight from an awareness of 'existential vacuum'—of boredom, ennui and meaninglessness.

Where such an interpretation is valid, the old saying, 'One is too many and a thousand never enough,' from the Alcoholics Anonymous Program, seems to apply very forcefully. Ultimately, however, it appears that only the discovery of meaning in life and of some form of self-transcendence, through creativity and contribution to others, can bring an authentic experience of empowerment, self-worth and enthusiasm for life. The individual who has made such a discovery is also necessarily more centred, inner-directed and less dependent upon powerful others for self-definition and affirmation. The person is now more of a master or mistress in his or her own house.

SOMA: SOCIETY OF MARVELLOUS ACCEPTANCE

If a key exists to a more enlightened way of understanding and caring in the AIDS area, it is likely to be discovered in a new vision or model, according to which HIV and its outcome reflect processes involving the total system of humans and their environment. This is an ecological or truly holistic concept of disease and healing—a concept I have called SOMA.

It embraces the whole person in its understanding of

disease as a process encompassing body, mind and spirit. I am using the word SOMA as an acronym for Society of Marvellous Acceptance (of self).

'Soma' is also the Greek word for the physical body. Thus the group 'body' represented by the letters S O M A, is made up of members who are learning to experience unconditional love and acceptance of themselves, including their bodiliness, sexuality, emotions and spirituality. Their quest is for wholeness and acceptance of all parts of themselves.

If this is the vision, what are the specific aims of SOMA, now and in the future?

The primary current aim of SOMA is to provide psychological means of therapy and healing for HIV antibody positive persons, their partners and families. SOMA does not duplicate services offered by other support groups or organizations.

The focus of individual and group work in SOMA is essentially upon the prevention of illness or the arrest of disease progression and the enhancement of the quality of life in HIV-infected people. In other words, the key aim is to facilitate change in those mental and spiritual factors shown by scientific research studies to be linked with immunity and disease, whether in HIV infection, cancer or other immune related illnesses.

A specific pattern of factors is relevant to both immunity and the onset and course of such illnesses. The pattern includes: a) repressed or bottled up emotions (anger); b) non-acceptance of gay identity; c) experiences of unresolved loss (death, separation, work); d) a sense of powerlessness over the outcome of HIV infection; e) hopelessness, giving up, or the 'curl up and die' response to diagnosis and f) lack of meaning or purpose in life.

All of these factors have been linked to immunity and disease by scientific studies and the links are statistically significant and powerful. What this means is that psychological methods (for example, individual and group therapy, creative visualization and meditation) can logically be expected to influence one's immune (T-cell) status and resistance to AIDS-related illness.

Clinical observation supports this bold and revolutionary claim. However, of course, proper trials, like those for AZT, are required to provide scientific validation. To date funding has been denied for such programs of research, perhaps because of the politics operating in the AIDS area (as one eminent professor has suggested in personal correspondence).

SOMA provides programs in the belief that against HIV we must use every tool and means of therapy, provided it has at least some scientific rationale. This is, I suspect, my own personal myth, or destiny, in Carl Jung's sense.

Because so many HIV-infected persons experience 'unfinished business' and difficulties with revealing their gay identity and health status to their families, SOMA provides appropriate counseling and support in this double 'coming out' process. Clinically, more than 95 per cent of the patients experience a quite marvellous process of reconciliation, healing and unconditional love with their families.

As more patients respond to therapy and realize inner growth by becoming involved with community groups such as CSN and Ankali, SOMA is becoming concerned with follow-up work, in the form of care for carers. This means addressing the need for programs which aim to prevent burn-out and to reduce stresses such as 'bereavement overload', following multiple deaths or loss experiences. Community support groups are especially vital in this area.

In the future, SOMA might well have a role to play in the provision and organization of such services as residential retreats, allowing for time out, stress reduction, and learning such coping skills as visualization and meditation for patients, partners, carers and families. However, this vision is at present in the realm of possibility only.

Perhaps an alternative vision of the AIDS epidemic is now needed. This could be the sharp and intense vision of the suffering face of Christ himself, in those who are sick, stigmatized, alienated and unchosen. It is the vision of Mother Teresa, who holds the suffering Christ in her arms, when she embraces the poor in the slums of Calcutta.

Several movements already exist within the churches, which could be considered as possible models of compassionate, outreach and ministry. These include such religious communities as the Servants of the Paraclete who provide residential and day-care programs for clergy and others suffering from stress burn out, alcoholism and crisis of vocation. The Taizé community is a model of an ecumenical approach to the problems of reconciliation and outreach, as well as formation in the religious life.

During the next decade, it is probable that the sheer magnitude of the global AIDS epidemic, affecting several million people, could call for the formation of dedicated movements or religious communities. Thus SOMA, in its current form, might well ultimately be subsumed or incorporated into a much larger whole, in the form of a religious movement which could possess the features outlined in the following section.

RELIGIOUS COMMUNITIES: MODELS AND STRUCTURES

Dedicated religious communities, ministering to marginalized people generally and in the HIV/AIDS area particularly, would be reconciling, healing and transformative in their essential functions. The members of such new communities would share a vision of the suffering face of Christ in all people to whom they ministered.

Such communities would need to possess a structure within which their members can experience authentic psychological support as well as nurture and nourishment in the spiritual life. Part of the miracle of Taizé, for example, aside from the awesome power, energy and vitality of its work in the areas of ecumenism and reconciliation, might well reflect the nourishment of the community through living symbol, sacrament and empowering liturgy.

With regard to the more specific type of model community being proposed here, a truly containing and supportive structure could integrate some or all of the following elements:

1. The creation of a core group of perhaps four to six people, who may choose to live and to work together in community, exercising their particular gifts in ministry. These individuals could be clergy, religious or lay people, who would commit to full or part-time work, for example, in the HIV/AIDS area and/or, for example, with homeless youth or with people with problems of alcoholism or other addiction.

2. The creation of another group of people, exercising a similar kind of ministry, but living separately, for example, married persons who are integrally part of the community, especially with respect to collective participation in the spiritual life—liturgy, sacraments, offices and other disciplines.

3. The spiritual life would become the centre of the community's shared experience of containment and empowerment, as well as agapean love. It would incorporate such disciplines and practices as the daily offices and Eucharist, devotion to the Blessed Sacrament, prayer, meditation, retreats and Taizé evenings or weekends.

4. Training, supervision and support for clergy, religious and lay people, working with bereavement, families, youth and persons living with HIV/AIDS. More specifically, all community members would be expected to have addressed and to have worked through their own attitudes towards mortality, loss, grief, human sexuality and attitudes towards minority or marginalized social groups. In certain areas of ministry, professional training would be an essential requirement.

The institution, during July 1991, of monthly healing services at St Joseph's Church, Newtown, in Sydney, represents perhaps a first step towards the formation of a religious community in the form we are describing. The services attempt to integrate the archetypal symbolic and sacramental dimensions of psychospiritual healing with scientific and professional approaches, such as counseling and psychotherapy.

Moreover, the healing services offer opportunities, through the use of ritual and symbol, for a collective and shared expression of grief, as well as the healing of painful memories and feelings. The services are conducted jointly by clergy, religious and lay people, who are experienced in work with persons who are coping with loss or living with HIV/AIDS. This group is already functioning, in a real sense, as a community.

For the 1991 World AIDS Day healing service, St Joseph's Church was filled, both with people and with a light, which seemed to be a symbol of the renewal and transformation of a parish that, like so many in inner-city areas, had appeared to be dying or even devoid of spiritual vitality. Many of the participants were people who were either alienated from mainstream churches or for whom this was a first experience of the rich treasures of Catholic liturgy and symbolic ritual.

During 1992, the plan is for the monthly healing services to become more formally integrated with a range of follow-up programs. This will include pastoral care, counseling, psychotherapy, welfare assistance and outreach to homeless, addicted and HIV infected youth as well as adults. Alcoholics Anonymous and Narcotics Anonymous will be invited to establish chapters, with the use of parish facilities.

Insofar as the church, in authentic imitation of Christ, strives, symbolically speaking, to feed those who are hungry for compassion, healing and meaning in their experience of darkness and suffering, it may itself be renewed by the discovery that many are drawn to participate in the liturgical and sacramental life. This is simply a re-finding of its timeless role and function, as a sacred, transformative space, within which reconciliation and healing can occur.

Finally, the members of an emerging community become the servants or instruments of this very process of reconciliation and healing. The story of the Curé d'Ars, who restored one of the most derelict parishes in the France of his day, might well be both a mirror and a source of inspiration with regard to this kind of process within the church.

For those whose theological positions may create doubts or scruples about the forms of community and ministry envisioned here, a reminder of the situation confronted by the infant church might well be timely. The sheer fact of historical distance, of course, may render it difficult for such people to imagine the enormity of the visible spiritual darkness in ancient Rome. However, saints Peter and Paul, among others, nevertheless carried the light of the resurrected Christ, like the paschal candle itself, into the very depths and heart, of that darkness.

Perhaps then, ministry to persons who are living with HIV/AIDS and at the very margins of our own society, could be construed not only as no less morally justifiable but also as an ultimate challenge to heroic, compassionate outreach and apostolate.

CHAPTER TWELVE

Spiritual Exercises with Archetypal Images and Symbols

This chapter begins with a series of exercises that make use of significant religious symbols—light and darkness, bread and wine, incense, oil and sacred icons. The exercises are intended first to enhance the bonding process in the therapeutic group and second to awaken authentic experiences of spirituality. This can be important for those—perhaps all in the group—who tend to be alienated from mainstream religion. This alienation usually reflects perceived homophobic attitudes within the churches as well as misogyny and personal trauma.

The religious symbols are presented in such a way as to facilitate the discovery (or recovery) of their unconscious meaning and psychospiritual significance, which integrates intellect and feeling, head and heart. And this process of inner integration or reconciliation is, I believe, vital to that real experience of wholeness which is the goal or quest of this whole book.

My own clinical experience is that the spiritual exercises outlined in this chapter induce powerful and moving experiences of this nature in people living with HIV/AIDS, or facing life-threatening illnesses.

Light and Darkness

This reflection is upon symbols and images which appear to be universal in their significance for the spiritual journey of humanity. The meaning and power of such symbols seem to be beyond the boundaries of both historic time and human culture. They are often called archetypal images and symbols, because of this universal, timeless quality.

(*Extinguish lights and ask participants to close their eyes*)

Let us reflect upon the symbols of darkness and light, which assume many forms, in terms of their psychic and spiritual significance. As a psychic image or symbol, darkness represents the state of *unconsciousness* and also all of those dimensions of the mind and spirit which exist as one's Shadow—the unknown, repressed, disowned and split-off wishes, tendencies and feelings, which we overlook or neglect. The deeper unconscious is also the source of our unrealized gifts, creativity and spirituality, including our unique personal meanings, destinies, dreams or 'myths', yet to be fulfilled in our lives.

The unconscious psyche already contains the answers to such questions as 'Why be?' and 'Why do I now not commit suicide—if I am truly facing a threat to life and if I have lost everything?'

Darkness also represents such mental states as loneliness, isolation, abandonment, despair, inner emptiness and meaninglessness (the 'dark night of the soul'), as well as death itself.

(*Light one central candle. One by one, light a candle or taper for each member of the group from the central candle*)

Now, when you are ready, open your eyes. Watch the circle of light slowly forming in the room. The light comes from a common source. As it is divided and distributed, passed from one person to another, the light, in creating a circle, gradually overcomes the darkness in the room, and perhaps also in your consciousness. Capture your feelings!

(*Pause*)

Light represents the expanding and deepening consciousness of one's self. It is an image of the goal or quest of one's inner journey or pilgrimage towards enlightenment, wholeness, integration and unity of the deeper self, as well as healing.

The inner journey or quest for enlightenment and wholeness is a theme of many myths and is central to the great religions of east and west, when viewed as pathways to full realization of the self or spirit, described in symbolic terms as nirvana or heaven in Buddhism and Christianity.

The deity, God image or central figure in such religions, is often represented as surrounded by a halo of light to suggest something of the energy, power and fascination of these role models of wholeness, enlightenment and self realization.

On a more personal or subjective level, the actual discovery and inner experience of the deepest self, and of wholeness, balance and harmony, is described by the saints and mystics in all of the great religious traditions in remarkably similar ways. All of these saints, mystics and gurus refer to images and experiences of the inner light. This light resembles a circular disc or sun, of indescribable beauty, often beginning as a point somewhere within the field of consciousness and spreading, filling the soul like some kind of luminous cloud.

The emotions and feelings one may feel are those intense joy, elation, ecstasy, lightness, energy and vitality, even of libido.

The means or pathways to such experiences include meditation and other spiritual exercises or disciplines, depending upon the religious tradition. These days, many patients pursuing deep psychotherapy, in certain forms, as well as by practicing meditation or creative visualization, experience very similar states to those described as 'enlightenment', wholeness or union with a God-Presence.

Perhaps, the circle of light forming in the room, beginning at a common source, then distributed among you, may have awakened feelings like those one can experience watching the sun rising, during a magnificent dawn, on a beach or mountain top. Such experiences are perhaps glimpses, hints and mirrors of an inner light, wholeness and well-being of even more sublime beauty and greater power which you may came to discern during your journey, in this group, as a member of SOMA.

This light, wholeness and love, can move through your being into all of your relationships, out and into the world—as if you are carrying and passing on a flame or torch.

Water

The equation, $E = mc^2$ represents, in abstract mathematical symbols, the fact that, under precise conditions, matter and energy are inter-changeable. Yet, the equation itself seems remote from the awesome reality of nuclear fission and the terrifying experience of an atomic explosion.

Religious creeds and dogmas are also, in a sense, abstract statements or representations of actual human experiences of the spiritual dimension of the psyche. Yet, as abstract formulas, they, like mathematical equations, seem very distant from *living* experiences of that inner wholeness, balance, harmony and ecstatic union with a deeper self or God-Presence, described by the saints and mystics of all ages and from the great religious traditions of east and west. St Thomas Aquinas, towards the end of his life, described the elaborate arguments of his *Summa Theologica* as 'so much straw' compared to the vision of God revealed by contemplation.

For many people, western religion has become unduly

cerebral, with a fatal imbalance in favour of the intellect. Belief in creeds and dogmas has tended to become a substitute for a form of knowing which embraces and fills the *whole* person. The decline of icons, images, symbolism and rituals since the Protestant Reformation has contributed to a dangerous neglect of feeling, intuition and sensory functions and to an over-valuation of intellect. Certain minds, of course, try to avoid and to defend themselves against real feeling, at almost any cost. Unfortunately, such people always tend to be suspicious of and to bear animosity towards those who no longer need to 'believe' because they *know* the presence of God, as a reality within and beyond themselves.

For the person who has it, a genuine religious experience is a priceless gift. As well as adding richness and meaning to one's life, it may even have a survival value. One of the aims of the type of psychotherapy you are experiencing here is to assist you in your search for a compelling meaning in life and in your quest for wholeness and healing of body, mind and spirit. The living religions of every age have always been the source of images and symbols which act as beacons or guiding lights on this inner journey.

We have already reflected upon the meaning of the symbols of darkness and light, as archetypal, timeless images, whose psychic or spiritual significance exists beyond the limits of human history and culture. We used the physical experience of the darkened room and lighted tapers as a practical means of grasping the symbols, so that what was happening externally might somehow mirror an inner reality. Tonight, we shall reflect briefly upon water as such a symbol or image with spiritual significance.

SYMBOLIC SIGNIFICANCE

Water appears as an image or theme in dreams, myths and many religious rituals. As a symbol, water might thus be compared to a river delta, with many tributaries or streams flowing from a common source and into an ocean of meaning which is eternal, limitless, infinite. In the following exercise in active-imagination water alludes to the psyche, the spirit or soul itself. Picture your own reflective-consciousness, the self, as resembling a bucket or urn of water.

Your experience of selfhood or identity, of being aware of being aware, may seem as if it is contained in such a vessel, which has boundaries, separating it from others and from the world. Now picture the bucket or urn of water being poured out into the ocean. Is the identity or continuity of the water contained in the vessel lost as it is poured out? Commonsense might suggest an immediate 'Yes' in answer to the question.

But in certain moments of awe, wonder, ecstasy, love and mystical experience of union with one's deeper self, something strange occurs. It is as if the boundaries of the vessel or container dissolve, but the integrity or unity of one's self is not only preserved but enhanced or strengthened. We face a paradox, that a remarkable heightening and strengthening of self and identity may occur through the very experience of boundary loss, union or fusion, in states of awe, wonder, joy, rapture and ecstasy. Such states can be induced, for example, by meditation, religious ritual, and, sometimes, by great music or art or making love.

Often, loss of the fear of death flows from peak or mystical experiences of the deeper self, Spirit or God-image. For the person is now moving away from a mere intellectual belief in a spiritual dimension, towards a deeper and more certain knowledge—that the personal identity or self possesses a continuity or *eternal* quality, which extends beyond irreversible brain-death. The deeper self is the butterfly, which will one day rise resplendent from the cocoon.

In the great religious traditions of east and west, water has many layers of symbolic meaning. Water is a symbol of initiation to sacred mystery, of spiritual awakening or rebirth, of rites of passage or transition from one stage in life to another. Myths embodying this type of meaning include the Parsifal legend or search for the Holy Grail, and the story of the Book of Exodus in the Old Testament, in which the Jews pass through the Red Sea, out of bondage, darkness and oppression under the Egyptians to a new freedom and identity.

Water baptism and the ritual tonsure or shaving of the head, in the Christian tradition, are symbolic representations and enactments of an inner process of spiritual rebirth, transformation and wholeness. The novice or newly-baptized person is said to have become 'a new creation', participating in a mystical or divine form of life or existence and to have become a child of God.

On a more practical level, water is a rich and powerful symbol of humility. This comes from being centred and in touch with the earth or ground of one's being, without arrogance, pretence or false pride. The spiritual attitude of humility is revealed in an openness and willingness to empty oneself out in loving service to others. The ritual washing of feet in the Christian Easter liturgy, is one example of the symbolic use of water in an enactment of humility and service. Through such loving service, one's living experience of inner transformation and wholeness is mirrored in action upon the world, in ways that touch the lives of others.

EXERCISE

We shall now try a bonding exercise using water as a symbol. During this brief exercise, we shall pass a bowl containing water around the group, three times.

(Each person has a cup, which they fill from the bowl)

As you receive the bowl for the first time, fill your cup, but please do not drink the water yet. Just reflect, as the bowl rests in your hands, and before passing it on, upon all of the *painful* memories, feelings, fears, hurts and resentments in your life—those you are aware of and those you may wish to avoid or to bury. Name them to yourself, or aloud if you prefer. Once you have called these painful memories, feeling and issues or concerns to mind, and named them, imagine that the cup now contains all of this fear, hurt and sorrow which you sense and feel within yourself. Pour the water from the cup back into the bowl—without drinking. You might each allow about thirty seconds to one minute to do all of this, before passing the bowl on to the next person—to do the same exercise.

(*Pause while group completes step one*)

Now let us repeat the exercise in a different way. This time, as you receive the bowl, fill your cup again. Now call to mind and reflect upon all of the *joyful* memories and feelings, you can recall—for example, experiences of holding, support, compassion, love and happiness—those you have had or wish for in the future. Name them to yourself, or aloud if you prefer. Now imagine, once more, that the cup is filled up with and contains all of this happiness, well-being and joy. Then, without yet drinking, pour the contents of the cup back into the bowl.

(*Pause while group completes step two*)

Now we shall pass the bowl around a third time. Again, fill your cup, then pass the bowl on to the next person, without drinking. When all have filled their cup from the bowl, drink the water you have in the cup.

As you drink the water, try to imagine that you are taking into yourself, all of the pain and all of the joy that was poured out into the bowl by the group members.

In this way, you are allowing yourself to participate, symbolically speaking, *as members of one body*, group or community, in each other's joys and sorrows, fears and hopes, and longings.

Through this sharing, you may also sense a cleansing or dissolving away of isolation, loneliness, darkness, feelings of being trapped, powerlessness or negativity. You may also experience some awakening of a sense of companionship and unanimity with those who are present.

Bread and Wine

In recent therapeutic sessions of this SOMA group, our focus during the reflections has been upon the nature and function of certain images and symbols which appear to be universal in their mental and spiritual significance. Such images are often called archetypal images because their meaning and fascination seem to extend beyond the boundaries of historic time and human culture. They function as beacons or guiding lights on humanity's spiritual journey towards inner wholeness and healing and in the quest for a compelling meaning or purpose in life.

Tonight, we shall reflect upon the symbolic significance of bread and wine, before moving on, next week, to some images and symbols which reflect the very substance of the psychotherapeutic process itself. A further bonding exercise may help to illustrate the practical function of symbols as a means of building a sense of identification and communion between the members of a spiritual or mystical 'body' or community.

This bonding exercise may serve another useful purpose. It also aims to show that certain external images and symbols, even when incorporated in ancient and traditional religious rituals are essentially 'mirrors' of, as well as a means of awakening, living spiritual experiences. These inner experiences are those of the deeper unconscious self, of wholeness and healing. These psychic experiences are often described as discoveries or encounters with a God-Presence within the person. This may assume the form of an inner light or 'vision', in dreams or in other altered states of consciousness, induced by meditation, visualization or religious liturgy.

Such psychic or spiritual experiences are always moving and the feeling states are typically those of awe, wonder, rapture, energy, elation and ecstasy.

BREAD

Let us now reflect upon bread as a symbol. As well as being a life-sustaining substance for the body, individually and collectively, bread means companionship, community, and sharing with others, as members of one body. It also represents the earth, the feminine and human production.

When a loaf of bread is broken, this symbolic act confronts us with a question, whenever we take part in a shared or community celebration of life, on both a spiritual plane as well as socially. This question is: How can one allow oneself to be taken, blessed or empowered, broken and distributed, like the bread, as a form of spiritual food for others? In other words, how can one become a holding, caring, sustaining and loving presence for others, those who are lost, empty, hungry for support, acceptance and unconditional love? This question applies especially to one's response to those who are angry, difficult, isolated or outcast—the 'unlovely'.

The 'breaking of bread' means a sacrificial emptying and offering of oneself through loving service to others—just as one is sustained spiritually by the 'food', the companionship, of one's membership in a 'mystical' body, whether that body is a church, a community or a therapeutic group like SOMA. Unfortunately, this symbolic meaning of the breaking of the bread in eucharist or communion often seems to have been lost in the lives of Christians, although Jesus himself put it at the very heart of the sacred mystery which he instituted.

EXERCISE

Let us now use the symbol of the breaking of bread in a brief bonding exercise.

(*A loaf of crusty bread in a basket is passed around the group*)

As the loaf is passed around, break off a small piece and hold it; without yet eating. As you hold the piece of bread, try to name aloud, or to yourself, something you really wish to change, or to become more fully conscious of, during your work in this SOMA group.

This something might, for example, be a Shadow quality or attitude that you are beginning to sense and to acknowledge within yourself. Examples are qualities such as fear, anger, hatred, insecurity, jealousy, hopelessness, powerlessness, loneliness, grief, lack of meaning or purpose, apathy or some burden or disappointment in your life.

Now put the piece of bread back into the basket, without eating any, and pass the basket on to the next person.

(*When all have broken the bread, pass the basket around again*)

This time, as you break off the piece of bread, take it and hold it. Reflect upon and then name aloud, or to yourself, one or more of the things you wish to change or to know better about yourself—how about self-centredness, or egoism or the tendency to manipulate others? Then, simply put the piece of bread into the basket, without eating, and pass it on to the next person.

(*When all have broken the bread, pass the basket around the group again. This time each person takes a piece of bread and eats it*)

We shall complete this symbolic exercise by actually eating the broken bread as it is distributed among us. In a symbolic way, we shall be taking into ourselves someone else's shadow, pain, problem or 'dis-ease'.

By eating the bread, we shall also be accepting some responsibility for supporting, holding and encouraging another person, through our participation in this group's work as members of the body of SOMA.

WINE

At a fundamental level, wine represents the psychic or spiritual energy and life shared by the members of a community or body, just as the branches of a vine are sustained and nourished by the sap flowing from a common source or rootedness. In certain religious traditions, wine is used to represent a symbolic giving of one's blood or life for others and as a ritual enactment of the surrender or sacrifice of one's ego to a deeper self and to a larger whole or community. The technical term for this process is 'self-transcendence', that is, overcoming egoism.

(*A cup of wine is passed around the group. Each person drinks from the cup*)

When the members of a group or community drink from the same cup, they participate symbolically in a sense of wholeness. As we pass the cup around in this SOMA group, try to reflect upon what this act of sharing means to you —in terms of your sense of belonging, identification and commitment to others.

One can have no greater love than that of emptying oneself and of laying down one's life for one's friends! How can *you* empty yourself of time, energy, presence and love, for others? How can you experience and realize genuine *agape* or spiritual love for others, for example, by sharing in the cup of their fear, loneliness, sadness and disease or in the cup of their experience of joy or the fulfilment of their dreams and meanings in life?

Incense: Celebrating and Remembering

'Let my prayer be counted as incense before you, and the lifting up of my hands, as an evening sacrifice' (Psalm 141).

Incense is a religious symbol with origins in the mists of history and its use is common to the spiritual traditions of both east and west. The ritual and symbolic use of incense probably began in primitive, animistic cultures as an element of sacrificial rites of expiation and fertility. In such animistic cultures, people lived in a state of 'projection', that is, they experienced unconscious parts of the psyche as deities or demons, which inhabited the external world. The evolution of religion consists, on one level, of the gradual dissolving and taking back of such psychic projections.

Thus, the 'twilight of idols' and the emergence of monotheism were steps in the process of an expansion and deepening consciousness of people's inner psyche or soul. They had begun to discover the 'kingdom of God' and the imprint of the divine within themselves. They had become in a symbolic sense 'children of God.'

The great religious traditions, then, function as channels of living symbols and as means of facilitating encounters with the God-image or Presence, as well as the deeper self. It is precisely this experience of the deeper self, spirit or God-image which is the purpose of humanity's symbolic rituals, liturgies and spiritual disciplines such as meditation.

At a primitive level, incense is a vestige of the idea of a sacrificial burnt offering, used in a rite of expiation or cleansing of collective guilt or Shadow qualities. Even at this rather archaic level, the rising smoke represents a spiritualization of matter, as the incense is burnt and transformed into an ethereal substance, ascending towards the 'sky-heaven', the dwelling-place of the deity.

On a more sophisticated and psychological level, the idea

of sacrifice tends to become the notion of surrender of one's ego to a higher power. Thus the incense retains its significance as an outward and visible sign of spiritual transformation and of a change of attitude, away from egoism and relative unconsciousness, towards a deeper enlightenment into and consciousness of one's inner psyche or self. This is one psychological meaning of the ritual censing of the altar during the Christian Mass or eucharist. And the underlying ideas of the spiritualization and transformation of matter, earth and the body still remain in the use of incense during funerals and other rites, at least in the Eastern Orthodox and Catholic traditions.

Many people with a Protestant background tend to experience an aversion to incense as well as to religious icons and symbols generally. This may, perhaps, be due to an over-evaluation of the purely rational, thinking side of human nature and to a one-sided neglect of sensation and feeling. However, another veiled concern might well be a fear of 'regression', that is, of being drawn back into a state of primitive projection, superstition and magical thinking or idolatry. For such people, a deeper psychological grasp of the meaning of religious symbols may be particularly helpful.

EXERCISE

Incense as a spiritual symbol is one means of celebrating and 're-member-ing' the presence of persons and figures who are, and have been, psychologically significant to us. We can actually use incense to help us, symbolically speaking, to hold or to call to mind such persons so that we may experience their presence, recapture or remember our feelings towards them. They may, perhaps, be people whom we have lost through death or separation and with whom we have some 'unfinished business' and need for reconciliation or forgiveness.

After a loss our grieving may be repressed, buried and

unresolved. Each loss in adult life tends to reawaken buried or unconscious memories and feelings about past experiences of loss and disappointment. One helpful, practical technique in working through loss and grief is the use in therapy of what are called 'linking objects'. Linking objects are items or things which remind us of lost persons who have died or from whom we have become separated or alienated. Examples of such objects are photographs, letters, items of clothing or other special things we shared with the loved person, like music or paintings.

(The group will have been asked beforehand to bring a linking object with them. A container of hot coals is placed in the centre of the group and another container of incense grains is passed around the group)

Let us now attempt a spiritual exercise using incense and relevant linking objects. First, we shall use two vessels; one containing hot coals, the other holding grains of fine incense. As the vessel containing the incense is passed around, take a few grains, then try to call to mind someone whom you have lost and whose presence you would like to experience. Perhaps you might ask this person to be present in some real way, which you can sense.

Now, reflect upon and name this person, pausing for a moment or two, just to listen, allowing yourself to capture your memories and feelings. When you are ready, take and hold the linking object (photograph, etc) to help remind you of this person. Capture whatever memories and feelings are awakened in your mind.

Then, once again, when you are ready, sprinkle the incense onto the hot coals in the vessel on the table. As the smoke rises, allow yourself to experience some sacred or precious moment or time you shared with the person whose presence you are now remembering.

When you have done this, pass the incense on to the next group member so that everyone completes the exercise. As this occurs, try to be still, to be silent, to capture whatever emotions and memories are awakened or surface within you.

Anointing with Oil, Healing Touch and Washing

'When he had washed their feet, Jesus said to the disciples, "Do you understand what I have done? I have given you an example, that you should do for one another what I have done for you"' (John 13:8–16).

When this incident occured, the group of twelve disciples had gathered in a secluded upper-room to celebrate the Jewish Passover. They were twelve very ordinary men, not at all like the figures of saintliness and otherworldliness often represented in stained glass or frescoes. In the beginning, they had probably been attracted to Jesus' extraordinary personal charisma. However, during his public ministry, Jesus no doubt became for his disciples a figure of truly archetypal, symbolic significance—as teacher, hero and ultimately, on the mountain of transfiguration, the longed-for saviour.

The incident of the washing of the disciples' feet therefore was a remarkable symbolic act, with profound relevance to their spiritual awakening, initiation and inner transformation. Such an act implied an attitude of deep humility, as washing feet was perhaps the most menial task, performed by servants in a Jewish household. It was also, in a tangible sense, an 'epiphany' or revelation of Jesus' own nature and spiritual significance to the world then and now.

In washing his disciples' feet, Jesus touched and engaged them in and through his human bodiliness and rootedness in the earth. He was revealing something of the mystery of his incarnation—he was truly God and truly human. He was also modeling the nature of their future bonding, as members of a 'mystical' body or community, held together by *agape*, that is, by spiritual love.

The spiritual awakening which was to occur in their collective consciousness at Pentecost would be described in such terms as a mighty, audible rushing of wind and as dancing tongues of fire—remarkably powerful manifestations of in-flowing, psychic energy. Such an experience appears to be truly archetypal in nature, transcending matter, space and time.

Let us now consider briefly the symbolic significance of such acts as touching, washing and anointing. These symbols appear in many religious traditions and rituals, in both east and west. They form a golden string of spiritual meaning running through human history. Such symbols occur as an integral part of rites of passage and transition, from one stage or form of life to another.

Ritual washing is an element of initiation to a sacred mystery and to membership in a mystical body or community. It is also a symbol of inner transformation and of the attitude of humility, necessary for participation in, or experience of, the God-image, or the deeper self, within and beyond the individual person.

Ritual anointing with oil is a symbolic element of such transitional experiences as preparation for death, the coronation and consecration of rulers and spiritual leaders, who will become the bearers or embodiments of both parental and divine images. Symbolic touching, holding and embracing also occur in such contexts as these, as well as being part of rites of healing and reconciliation.

Pope Innocent III became so alarmed by the emotions and 'unruly' passions sometimes awakened by ritual holding, embracing and kissing, that he removed such dangerous practices from the celebration of the Mass—once known as an *agape* or spiritual love feast. These elements have only recently been restored.

What might be the psychic functions of such symbolic or ritual acts of touching, washing and anointing? On one level, of course, they tend to affirm that very bodiliness and rootedness in the earth shared by all people and which form a powerful basis for human identification and bonding.

Touch itself is perhaps the most primitive means of both providing and expressing mutual holding, acceptance, reconciliation and love between the members of a group, body or community. The absence of adequate experience of holding early in life results in emotional crippling, stunted growth and impoverishment of the personality. Secondly, touch, in its various symbolic forms, is one vital means of facilitating the process of identification, bonding and participation in a group or community. Through touch, barriers, defences and 'body armour' tend to dissolve and the experience of *agape* or spiritual love can be enhanced.

Thus, if the members of a group can all, symbolically speaking, allow themselves to wash one another's feet, then they may be lifted up and out of their egoism and isolation. They may also discover some of the many faces of that joy which flows from loving service and ministry to others—especially those who experience themselves as unlovely and untouchable because of exposure to HIV.

EXERCISE

Now we shall attempt a brief spiritual exercise, using symbolic touch and a form of anointing with oil. The whole exercise is best carried out in complete silence so that the group members can get in touch with their sensations and feelings.

Each person present will work with one partner, massaging with oil first the feet and then the hands of the other, for a few moments according to signals which I shall give. Then, I shall ask you to reverse roles; so that everyone experiences the massage and anointing.

As you complete the exercise, try to capture, in the silence, your feelings, simply acknowledging what they are, without as yet naming or openly expressing them. You will, of course, have ample opportunity to express such feelings and to discuss what the experience meant to you a little later.

The aim of the exercise is to help to expand and to deepen your consciousness of yourselves as members of this group, sharing common goals, meanings and purposes. It may also help to facilitate the growth of group spirit among us—a community of souls made in the image of God and capable of experiencing the God present within and beyond us.

When the group anointing is complete, the leader washes the feet of those present. In this way, he or she acts as a living icon of Christ's presence, compassion and unconditional love, for all people, even those who are despised, stigmatized, outcast and judged by others. As Jesus said, concerning the woman, 'Her sins, which are many, are forgiven, because she loved much!'

THE LAYING ON OF HANDS

Another ancient symbolic and ritual practice which utilizes touch is that of the laying on of hands. This rite is common during liturgies of healing within the mainstream churches and its deeper meaning can be grasped more fully in situations which allow the symbol to be re-presented in a way that is both human and refreshing, for example, in small groups.

The following exercise is one which I have found to be moving and powerful in group psychotherapy. The group members work in pairs. The instructions are that first one partner of each pair will stand facing the other, who stays seated. Full eye-contact is maintained for a moment, in complete silence, then the person who is standing lays both hands upon the head and later the shoulders of the other, allowing perhaps up to one minute for each body part or step.

According to a signal given by the therapist or group facilitator, the partners then reverse roles. Before the exercise actually begins, the group leader should try to focus the experience with several of the following orienting remarks or suggestions:

(a) As you allow yourselves to touch and to be touched, capture your feelings. Perhaps, you will sense a gentle dissolving away of boundaries or separateness.

(b) You may experience the washing away, cleansing or lightening of heavy, negative emotions like shame or guilt.

(c) Perhaps you will gradually become aware of rippling, glowing feelings of warmth, care and loving energy—or a sense of empowerment.

Finally, the group members are told that they will be able to discuss their experiences after the exercise is completed. The importance of maintaining silence during the actual exercise is to be emphasized, so that the experience within the person is as vivid and intense as possible on the levels of sensation and feeling. The exercise can be completed with a group experience of the ritual *embrasio* or hug, which symbolically represents the exchange of peace and reconciliation between people who are acknowledging and becoming conscious of their human, Shadow qualities and attitudes.

The Use of Icons

Religious icons are a symbolic means of representing the many faces of both the deeper self and the God image within the individual and collective human psyche. In fulfilling this symbolic function, icons can facilitate the processes of expanding and deepening our consciousness of the archetypal images they reflect. They act as beacons or guiding lights for the inner journey, the pilgrimage to healing.

The effective use of icons in spiritual exercises and meditation depends very much upon the attitude with which we approach them. It is similar to the attitude we might take towards great music or any other art.

This attitude is essentially one of complete openness and receptiveness, involving the suspension of judgement, expectation and purely rational thought. We become, in other words, like little children, humble, with a vision cleansed of prejudice and fear, in order to enter the 'kingdom of heaven', the spiritual dimension, within ourselves.

An enlightened, practical use of religious icons during meditation need not imply idolatry or superstition. Idolatry and superstition consist of a regressive or primitive misuse of such things, as if they are fetish objects or talismans, to which magical properties are attributed. This may be observed sometimes in the use of rosary beads or scapulars by certain Catholics who have not yet grasped the real meaning of symbols.

The icon, as a symbol, points beyond itself to a deeper, transcendent reality within and beyond the person. It functions as an instrument or channel of authentic religious experience by creating a medium or bridge between the outward sense (visible sign) and inner psychic reality, which may be later translated into theological language. What is essential is the living experience itself, in contrast to the purely intellectual grasp or statement of it. Authentic religious or mystical experience embraces the whole person—head and heart, intellect and feeling—in its powerful mystery and numinosity.

The selection of specific icons as focuses of meditation must always reflect a deep sensitivity to peoples' diverse religious backgrounds and aesthetic values. It is also wise to comment upon or clearly amplify the archetypal or universal significance of the image, represented by a particular icon, in humanity's collective experience of the deeper self or God image. This can be done by using cross-cultural examples of how the symbols or figures of 're-birth', the 'mother', the 'hero' and the 'saviour' have been manifested throughout human history; both in religion and in popular myth.

Icons created during the Byzantine and Baroque periods, for example those described in the delightful book, *Behold the Beauty of the Lord: Praying with Icons*, seem to work well, in terms of both aesthetics and rich, symbolic meaning. The twelfth century Virgin of Vladimir and Rublev's fifteenth century icon of the Saviour are particularly beautiful representations of key Christian mysteries and archetypal themes.

EXERCISE

Once the icon to be used as the focus of a meditation has been chosen, it should be placed in a central location in the room, for example, on a chair, table or altar. It should be well illuminated, perhaps by lighted tapers or candles. For very large rooms an overhead slide of the icon may be preferable.

STEP ONE consists of instructions which aim to induce very deep relaxation by means of breathing exercises, like those described in chapter eleven. These exercises are identical to those used for creative visualization or for meditation generally.

STEP TWO consists of cues and instructions about how to focus upon the features and symbolic qualities as well as the 'mystery' or spiritual meaning of the icon. A connection is established between the outward sense or image and an inner experience of it, for the person who is meditating. The following instructions will illustrate how such a connection might be created in a way which I have found to be effective in group work.

'Open your eyes, now that you are breathing freely and deeply and relaxed, and focus upon the face of the figure represented in the icon. Simply take in the form, contours, shape, colour and texture through your senses, so that an inward vision can begin to unfold. Close your eyes for a moment, then slowly open them again. Once more, focus upon the face, noting any subtle changes which may occur in form or movement or expression, as the figure is illuminated by or revealed to your consciousness.

'Close your eyes again for a few moments, then open them again, this time focusing only upon the eyes. Try to sense into whom or into what space and time the eyes are looking. Hold your gaze into the eyes, without blinking, for a while. Where are you in relation to the eyes, and where they are focused or looking?

'Close your eyes again, just resting quietly for a few moments. Now open your eyes, focusing upon the expression in the eyes and face of the figure represented in the icon. Try to sense the feelings expressed, especially by the eyes, as you focus your gaze, without blinking as far as possible.

'Perhaps you are beginning to sense and feel within yourself peace, sadness, love or great compassion, somehow mirroring the expression in the eyes and face of the figure which you are focusing upon. Just allow whatever happening to unfold, to continue as it is. Close your eyes for a while, simply being still, sitting with the experience.

'Open your eyes again, this time taking in the whole icon or figure, moving from the eyes and face, sensing the total form, the contours and details of the body. Allow the image as a whole to fill your consciousness and to touch your soul, with whatever meaning or spiritual mystery it possesses for you, at this moment, in the here and now. Perhaps you will also experience some illumination into the humanness and closeness of this figure—as a presence, within and beyond you.

'Close your eyes, be still and silent, as if you have just gazed through a kind of window into eternity—into a deep and timeless sacred space within your self.

STEP THREE consists of group discussion of the experience, preferably after a few minutes of complete silence.

Concluding Comments

This example of the use of religious icons in meditation concludes chapter twelve and its description of practical spiritual exercises for group therapeutic work. Those who choose to use such pathways to spiritual awakening and to the discovery of the deeper self, may find that they themselves are personally challenged to live the timeless 'mystery' in their own ministry and practice in the HIV/AIDS field and pastorate. To do this means becoming living icons of Christ's own presence, offering unconditional love and compassion—even in the darkest moments and places.

Finally, in principle, all of the spiritual exercises described in this chapter could be incorporated into intensive workshops and retreats for people living with HIV/AIDS, as well as for their families and carers. Insofar as these exercises do, in fact, employ spiritual symbols, whose meaning appears to be truly archetypal or universal in nature, they might well contribute something, however small, to the process of renewal and transformation within the churches themselves, even at the level of seminary training and formation of priests and ministers. This transformative process is something that is already revealed in such ecumenical movements as that of Taizé.

POSTSCRIPT

A Dream of Gerontius

I wish to conclude this book by communicating the content of a dream. I have named it after a poem by John Henry Newman. The dream occured after a session of therapy with a dying patient, whom I shall refer to as 'Gerontius', Newman's poetic figure.

Gerontius was experiencing a process of accelerated spiritual growth, even as his cancer had begun to spread, consuming him from within. His discovery of a God-image or presence, as a dimension of his deeper self, was accompanied by some quite extraordinary dreams, visions and mystical states of joy, elation and even of ecstasy. He was now experiencing spiritual healing and inner wholeness, in spite of the gradual disintegration of his body.

As I shared Gerontius' inner pilgrimage, I became acutely aware of the many other thousands of people who would probably never receive even the crumbs of such a spiritual banquet. The dream illustrates the grave problem of providing proper psychospiritual and pastoral care to all those who live with HIV/AIDS.

As the dream began, I found myself caught up in a stream of music, of sublime and ineffable beauty, majesty and power. The music resembled nothing I had ever heard. Slowly I started to experience the sound as if it had become a light or radiance, which surrounded and enveloped me. I sensed an upwards movement, like a form of levitation, as if I was leaving my body.

From somewhere within the light which resembled a cloud, an image appeared. It assumed the form of a Byzantine Christ, as if an icon of this period had somehow materialized. But the figure now standing before me was clearly a living one, awesome in its intensity and presence. This figure was clothed in vestments, though definitely not the traditional ones of the church's year. The vestments were of a replendent blue and gold and the Byzantine figure radiated a remarkable energy and power.

I experienced a voice, as if the dream-figure was now addressing me personally, in deep and resonant tones. The actual words were:

> 'My image is continually lost, century after century. It must be discovered and renewed, in people's hearts, in every age, until the end of earthly time!'

I now found myself, whether out of the body or floating or levitating, in a vast space like an infinite sphere, feeding a kind of sacramental bread to a seemingly endless sea of faces, stretched out around me. Some of the faces I vaguely recognized, others I did not yet know. I awoke with a feeling of incredible energy and vitality, yet also sadness that the dream-vision was already beginning to recede.

How might such a strange dream be interpreted, given the context in which it occurred?

On one level, of course, it could be understood simply as an expression of a powerful countertransference, that is, of an unconscious identification and emotional response to my dying patient. His unconscious, symbolic significance to me would have been represented by the dream appearance of a kind of 'saviour' figure. Perhaps, too, I had an unconscious wish to be a saviour for this remarkably gifted patient!

Alternatively, one might ask who or what else the dream figure was, whether a self-representation or something else. Who had I found myself holding and accompanying towards the consummation of his life and its final transition?

The dream, occuring in apparent synchronicity with Gerontius' real experience of spiritual healing, could have a deeper archetypal significance and concern some form of meaning or personal myth, yet to be fulfilled, in my own life. Whether such an interpretation is correct is a matter for others to assess in retrospect!

That the dream also contains and expresses an underlying theme of challenge to the churches, as well as to society in general, is something of which I can be much more certain. This challenge is consistent with Newman's own dream and prophetic vision and it is about renewal, transformation and a mission to reach out to the very margins of society, to all those who are hungry, outcast, stigmatized and in spiritual darkness, because they are now living with HIV/AIDS.

However, this process of reaching out must be with attitudes of genuine humility and absolutely unconditional love, acceptance and compassion, and whatever movements arise in this process must be practical, addressed to real human need and suffering. If collectively we ignore the challenge, we may eventually hear the words expressed in Matthew's gospel (25: 31–46):

> 'Depart from me ... for I was hungry and you gave me no food, thirsty and you gave me no drink, a stranger and you did not welcome me, naked and you did not clothe me, sick and in prison and you did not visit me ... As you did it not to the least of these, you did it not to me!'

APPENDIX

Presenting Patients: What to Look for and How

These notes are written primarily for counselors and community carers beginning work with HIV-infected persons, rather than for experienced clinicians. They are intended to illustrate some of the significant things to look for and how to look for them, in assessing presenting patients after diagnosis of HIV antibody positive status or symptoms of AIDS spectrum illnesses.

An enhanced ability to recognize these sorts of psychological factors and processes will promote empathy and effectiveness. The importance of knowing when to refer patients for professional help and of training and supervision has already been emphasized in this book.

The assessment guide provided here is a summary of a more technical outline of the use of behavioural techniques for identifying defense mechanisms and emotional states in persons with symptoms of malignancy that was published in the *British Journal of Medical Psychology* in 1978. In this paper, I describe the use of behavioural criteria for the rating of such factors by multiple trained observers, assessing video tape recorded interviews with patients. The results indicated that such methods were both reliable and valid in predicting relevant behaviour.

Bottled-up Anger

One common clue to the presence of repressed or bottled-up anger or rage is found in patients' responses to the request, 'Tell me about your last experience of being angry'. Persons who characteristically repress negative emotions and who are out of touch with their emotions will often deny any ability to recall such an experience, even for periods extending back several years!

Individuals less severely prone to using denial or repression as defenses against threatening realities, including feelings, will display observable discrepancies between verbal self-reports, what they say, and their non-verbal or 'body-language' responses. Thus, when describing situations which would be expected to arouse anger or resentment, they may not acknowledge verbally feelings which seem obvious from their posture, facial expressions and reports of symptoms such as pulse rate, stomach upsets or headaches.

Another helpful technique is to listen carefully to patients' descriptions of fantasies and dreams which include aggressive material. Many persons who find their own feelings of anger or rage frightening or unacceptable attribute these emotions and motives to others. Typically, these individuals report feeling that others (doctors, nurses, partners) are angry with them or express a preoccupation with other peoples' 'destructiveness'. The extreme manifestion of this use of projection is, of course, a paranoid attitude.

Depression

Depression can be inferred from statements indicating hopelessness, helplessness, worthlessness, shame and guilt. The pervasive feelings are of giving up or a sense of being disappointed in the ability of significant others to supply support, to boost self esteem or even magically to rescue patients from their troubles.

Examples of statements revealing these sorts of feelings are: 'It's useless.' 'Life isn't worth living any more.' 'I've lost interest in things around me.' 'I don't care what happens to me.' 'Who cares whether I'm around or not?' 'What's the use of asking for help?' 'No-one needs me any more.' 'I'm a failure.' 'It's degrading for me.' 'I feel silly (stupid, ashamed).' 'Like this, I'm of no use to my partner or anyone else.' 'I wish I hadn't been so angry (with the doctor, my partner).' 'I should have heeded the advice about safe sex.' 'AIDS is to me a terrible punishment.' 'I wish I was straight, because then I wouldn't have this filthy disease.'

Masked Depression

Persons who are repressing or masking symptoms of depression present a problem, even for experienced clinicians. Such people may appear, on the surface, to be in emotional equilibrium or even to be quite happy. However, such responses may conceal underlying depression or a decision to attempt suicide.

One effective way of picking up a state of masked depression, is to ask the question, 'Why would you not commit suicide?'

Persons who cannot answer the question at all or who stammer out hollow or phony replies are usually covering up feelings of depression and may be at risk for a suicide attempt.

A history of such self-destructive behaviours as drug and alcohol abuse is another significant clue to the presence of depression, often reflecting unresolved grief and inward-turning anger or rage.

Repression and Denial

Persons using the defenses of denial and repression usually present with bland emotions and make characteristic statements implying deliberate attempts to avoid thinking about the sources of threat implicit in the situation of facing screening for HIV antibody status or diagnosis of symptoms. The extreme use of such avoidance defenses may also result in delayed presentation with symptoms or not seeking medical advice at all, as well as presenting with other health problems, with a covert fear that these might reflect HIV infection.

Typical statements include: 'I don't want to think about it.' 'I put it out of my mind.' 'I couldn't have AIDS because I am so physically fit.' 'I didn't believe that I could have been infected because my partner was so clean and healthy-looking.' 'I'm not worried. My family's medical record is perfect.'

Disowned Sexual Identity

Many patients have never fully accepted or integrated a positive sense of homosexual identity or may, in response to diagnosis, regress to earlier stages of homosexual identity formation. Attentive listening during interviews reveals negative statements about homosexuals, representing a projection of self-hating or homophobic attitudes. Such statements include apparently joking references to other homosexual men as queens, 'faggots', 'poofters' and so on. Expressions of guilt, shame or regret about one's homosexuality will be obvious. In more extreme cases of 'egodystonic' homosexuality, patients may be overtly suicidal or self-destructive.

More subtle symptoms of split-off or disowned sexual identity include attempts to 'pass as straight', so that sexual behaviour is dissociated from the rest of the person's personal life and experienced anonymously and casually. Sometimes excuses are offered, such as: 'I am having problems with my wife.' 'I can't find an attractive woman.' 'I was drunk.'

Situational homosexuality, of course, exists, for example in jails or at sea, but such men usually prefer heterosexual partners when they are available.

Locus of Control

The concept of locus of control refers to a person's belief that life events or health status reflect external factors, such as fate or the influence of powerful others, or internal factors, such that the individual feels responsible for what happens.

Persons whose locus of control is *external*, will attribute outcomes to fate, chance or powerful others, such as doctors. Typical statements include: 'What happens to me is in the hands of my doctor.' 'I am powerless over what happens, now that I am antibody positive.' 'The doctor said there is a good chance I will get seriously ill, so there is little I can do—we are helpless.' 'I'll just have to sit back and hope for the best'.

Persons with an *internal* locus of control, on the other hand, will make statements like: 'I'm not going to hold on to the doom and gloom, I'm going to change my diet and do some meditation classes.' 'I'm going back to the gym and I want to work in a group on changing my attitudes.' Having an *internal* locus of control is linked with a better prognosis in a range of illnesses.

Existential Vacuum

The survivors of the Nazi concentration camps, as well as cancer and AIDS, have taught us that the spiritual dimension of meaning or purpose in life is vital to overcoming such extreme human conditions and life-threatening illnesses. When we discover a purpose or meaning in life, we have something or someone to live for and we possess a fighting spirit. The 25,000 recorded cases of near-death experiences all testify to the importance of having 'unfinished business'—tasks or goals to complete or a sense of personal myth and destiny—to survival.

However, many patients, perhaps the majority, diagnosed as HIV antibody positive or as having AIDS-related illnesses are caught in what is called an 'existential vacuum'. This is a state in which people experience an inner void or emptiness, characterized by a sense of meaninglessness and a lack of a purpose, goals and direction in life. Often the existential vacuum is covered up by patterns of behaviour, especially addiction to drugs, alcohol or impersonal sex, which create a sense of numbness or oblivion. Individuals may appear to be having a good time, but their emotional and spiritual life is shallow and impoverished.

Psychotherapy, meditation and creative visualization are usually necessary to help such people discover a sense of spirituality, meaning and purpose, as well as a renewed will to live. This dimension of the healing process is generally one of the most confronting and yet it is perhaps the most vital to survival.

BIBLIOGRAPHY

Ader, R., *Psychoneuroimmunology*, Academic Press, New York, 1981.
Alexander, F., *Psychosomatic Medicine*, Norton, New York, 1950.
Bartrop, R.W., 'Depressed Lymphocyte Function after Bereavement', *The Lancet*, 1977, 1, 834–836.
Bahnson, C.B., 'Stress and Cancer: State of the Art', *Psychosomatics*, Part 1, 1980, 21, 975–981; Part 2, 1981, 22, 207–220.
Camus, A., *The Myth of Sisyphus*, Hamish Hamilton, London, 1973.
Cass, V., 'Stages in Homosexual Identity Formation and the Coming Out Process', *Journal of Homosexuality*, 1979.
Cooley, W.W. & Lohnes, P.R., *Multivariate Data Analysis*, Wiley, New York, 1971.
Crisp, A.H., 'Psychosomatic Aspects of Neoplasia', *British Journal of Medical Psychology* 1970, 1, 175.
Delmonte, M.M., 'Physiological Concomitants of Meditation Practice', *International Journal of Psychosomatics*, 1984, 31(4), 23–26.
Engel, G.L., 'Memorial Lecture: the Psychosomatic Approach to Individual Susceptibility to Disease', *Gastroenterology*, 1974, 67, 1085–1093.
Engel, G.L., 'The Need for a New Medical Model: A Challenge for Biomedicine', *Science*, 1977, 196, 129–136.
Fox, B., 'Psychosocial Factors in Neoplasia: Studies in Man', in *Psychoneuroimmunology*, R. Ader (ed), Academic Press, New York, 1981.
Frankl, V.E., *Man's Search For Meaning: An Introduction to Logo-therapy*, Hodder & Stoughton, London, 1964.
Frankl, V.E., *Psychotherapy and Existentialism*, Souvenir Press, London, 1967.
Frankl, V.E., *The Unheard Cry for Meaning*, Washington Square Press, 1985.
Freud, S., *The Interpretation of Dreams*, George Allen & Unwin, London, 1966.
Freud, S., *The Psychopathology of Everyday Life*, Ernest Benn, London, 1966.
Fromm, E., *The Sane Society*, Routledge & Kegan Paul, London, 1963.

Greer, S. & Morris, T., 'Psychological Attributes of Women Who Develop Breast Cancer: A Controlled Study', J. Psychosomatic Research 1975, 19, 153.
Grinker, R.R., *Psychosomatic Concepts*, Jason Aronson, New York, 1973.
Illich, I., *The Nemesis of Medicine*, London, 1972.
Jacoby, M., *Individuation and Narcissism*, Routledge, London and New York, 1990.
Jemmott, J.B. & Locke, S.E., 'Psychosocial Factors, Immunologic Mediation and Human Susceptibility to Infectious Diseases: How Much Do We Know?', *Psychiatric Bulletin*, 1984, 95(1), 78–108.
Jung, C.G. *The Archetypes and the Collective Unconscious*, Routledge, London, 1990.
Jung, C.G., *Psychology and Religion: West and East*, Routledge & Kegan Paul, London, 1958.
Kissen, D.M., 'Psychosocial Factors, Personality and Lung Cancer in Men Aged 55–64', *British Journal of Medical Psychology*, 1967, 40, 29–43.
Klecka, W.R., 'Discriminant Analysis', in *Statistical Package for the Social Sciences*, Second Edition, Nie, N.H. et al (eds), McGraw Hill, New York, 1970.
Kübler-Ross, E., *AIDS: The Ultimate Challenge*, MacMillan, 1989.
Kuhn, T.S., *The Structure of Scientific Revolutions*, 1970.
Kutz, I. 'Meditation As An Adjunct to Psychotherapy: An Outcome Study', Psychother. Psychosom., 1985, 43, 209–218.
Lazarus, A.A., *Behavior Therapy and Beyond*, McGraw Hill, New York, 1971.
Levy, S.M., 'Prognostic Risk Assessment in Primary Breast Cancer by Behavioral and Immunologic Parameters', *Health Psychol.* 1985, 4(2), 99–113.
Locke, S.E. et al, *Foundations of Psychoneuroimmunology*, Aldine, New York, 1985.
Magarey, C.J. & Todd, P.B. 'Psychosocial Factors Influencing Delay and Breast Self Examination in Women with Symptoms of Breast Cancer', *Social Science & Medicine*, 1977, 11, 229–232.
Magarey, C.J. & Todd, P.B., 'Breast Loss and Delay in Breast Cancer Diagnosis—Behavioural Science in Surgical Research', *Australian and New Zealand Journal of Surgery*, 46, 391–393.
Magarey, C.J., 'Meditation—The Essence of Health', in *Inner Healing*, Drury, N. (ed), Harper & Row, Sydney, 1985, 132–144.
Magarey, C.J., 'Healing and Meditation in Medical Practice', *Medical Journal of Australia*, 1981, 1, 338–341.
Marmor, J., *Homosexual Behavior: A Modern Reappraisal*, Basic Books, New York, 1980.
Maslow, A.H., *Motivation and Personality*, Harper & Row, New York, 1954.
Maslow, A.H., *The Psychology of Science: A Reconnaissance*, Harper & Row, New York, 1966.
Menninger, K., *Man against Himself*, Harcourt, Brace, New York, 1938.

Medical Journal of Australia, AIDS Issue, October, 1984.
Nagel, E., *The Structure of Science: Problems in the Logic of Scientific Explanation*, Routledge & Kegan Paul, London, 1971.
Nemiah, J.C., 'Psychology and Psychosomatic Illness; Reflections on Theory and Research Methodology', Psychother. Psy-chosom. 1973, 22, 106–111.
Popper, K.R., *The Logic of Scientific Discovery*, Hutchinson, London, 1972.
Schmale, A.H., 'Hopelessness as a Predictor of Cervical Cancer', *Social Science & Medicine*, 1971, 5, 95–100.
Schleifer, R.W., 'Bereavement and Lymphocyte Function', Paper presented at the American Psychiatry Association, May, 1980.
Silverstein, C., *Man to Man: Gay Couples in America*, William Morrow & Co. New York, 1981.
Solomon, G.F. & Amkraut, A.A., 'Psychoneuroendocrinological Effects upon the Immune Response', Annual Review of Microbiology, 1981, 35, 155–184.
Solomon, G.F., 'Emotional and Personality Factors in the Onset and Course of Autoimmune Diseases: Particularly Rheumatoid Arthritis', in Ader, R. (ed) *Psychoneuroimmunology*, Academic Press, New York, 1981.
Solomon, G.F., 'Psychoimmunity of Long-Survivors of HIV Infection,' *Annuals of New York Academy of Science*, 1987.
Teilhard de Chardin, P., *The Future of Man*, Collins, London, 1964.
Todd, P.B. & Magarey, C.J., 'Ego-Defences and Affects in Women with Breast Symptoms: A Preliminary Measurement Paradigm', *British Journal of Medical Psychology*, 1978, 51, 177–189.
Todd, P.B., 'Cancer Education: A Copernican Revolution', *Cancer Forum*, 1974, 1, 8–11.
Todd, P.B., Burcham, J. et al. 'Psychosocial Factors Predicting HIV Antibody Status, T-Cell Immunity and Symptoms of AIDS Spectrum Disorders', in *Consultation on Psychology and Preventive Health*, Australian College of Clinical Psychologists, 1988.
Todd, P.B., 'Psychosocial Interventions in HIV Infection: A Preliminary Report on Progress with Group Counselling and Visualization', in *Consultation on Psychology & Preventive Health*, Australian College of Clinical Psychologists, 1988.
Todd, P.B., Harvey, I. & Powell, C., 'Christianity and Psychology: A Rapprochement?' *Australian Psychologist*, November 1987.
Winnicott, D.W., *Psychoanalytic Explorations*, Karnac Books, London, 1989.

INDEX OF TOPICS

aggression, 3
anger, 13, 16, 22, 24, 26, 33, 34, 36, 39, 40, 41, 42, 51, 61, 72, 75, 77, 96, 97, 108, 141–2

burn out, 3, 46–7, 68

cancer, 5, 15, 21, 108, 138
   denial of, 99
   emotional and psychological factors and, 12–14, 16, 25–6, 51, 60, 70, 96
   meditation and, 86
   visualization and, 53
countertransference, 3, 42, 45–6, 139

denial, 13, 22, 33, 60, 72, 99–101, 103, 143
depression, 3, 13, 15, 16, 24, 32, 33, 34, 39, 40, 60, 72, 75, 96, 97, 142–3

education programs, 60–3

fundamentalism, 62, 93–4, 102

germ theory, see medical model
groups
   exercises, 4, 114–37
   therapy, 2, 13, 39, 43, 50–2, 60, 77–8, 81, 97–8, 108

healing, vi, vii, 2–3, 5, 6, 44, 90, 105
   communities of, 110–13
   light and, 116
   meditation and, 52–5
   spirituality and, 19, 138, 140
   touch, 130
   visualization and, 43, 52–5, 84–6
holism, 4, 14, 15, 18, 19–20, 31, 107–8
homophobia, 6, 39, 61, 73–4, 76, 95–8, 100, 102, 114

homosexual identity, 2, 32, 33, 35–6, 39, 61, 81, 96, 97, 108, 143–4
  formation of, 63, 72–4, 91–4
  group support in, 51, 77
  mirroring and, 41, 45

loss, 13, 16, 22, 23–4, 32, 33, 34, 39, 40, 45, 51, 74, 75, 77, 96–7, 101, 108, 127–8
love, 55, 67, 73, 75–7, 78, 85, 88, 89, 92–3, 104, 111, 119, 120, 121, 123, 125, 131–2, 133, 136

meaning
  sense of, 18–19, 24, 39, 43, 46–51, 54, 68–70, 96, 98, 108–9, 122, 144–5
medical model, 5, 9–10, 11, 14
meditation, 39, 42–3, 52–3, 60, 81, 86–8, 98, 108–9, 116, 117, 123, 134–6, 145
mid-life crisis, 106

psychoneuroimmunology, 2, 13, 16, 21, 25, 27, 32, 39, 47–8
psychosomatic medicine, 2, 15, 16, 17, 25

repression, 13, 16, 22, 32, 73, 98, 101–4, 108, 141–3

screening, 3, 59–60, 99
sexuality, 2, 16, 55, 62–3, 66–7, 71–8, 102, 104–7
specificity hypothesis, 22–3
spirituality, 3–4, 6, 19, 53–5, 68–9, 81, 86–8, 106–7, 110–13, 114
  exercises, 114–37
symbols, vi, 4, 54, 94, 110, 112, 118, 114–37
  archetypal, 69, 87, 115, 118, 122, 133–5

T-cell, 13, 26, 31, 32, 33, 34, 36, 43, 60, 99, 108

visualization, 13, 39, 42–3, 52–3, 60, 81–6, 88, 108, 117, 123, 145